Avicenna On Diagnosis Signs and Symptoms

Adapted By

Laleh Bakhtiar

From Translations by
O. Cameron Gruner and Mazar H. Shah
Correlated with the Arabic by Jay R. Crook
with Notes by O. Cameron Gruner

Great Books of the Islamic World, Inc.

Printed in the United States of America.

Library of Congress Cataloging-in-Publication Data

Ibn Sina, Abu Ali al-Husayn ibn Abd Allah
The Canon of Medicine (al-Qanun fi'l tibb)
Lecture 11 - On Diagnosis Signs and Symptoms
1. Islam. 2. Medicine. I. Title

ISBN 10 (Book): 1-56744-789-9
ISBN 13 (Book): 978-1-56744-789-7
ISBN 10 (eBook): 1-56744-790-2
ISBN 13 (eBook): 978-1-56744-790-3

Cover Design by Liaquat Ali
Cornerstones are Allah and Muhammad connected by Bismillah al-Rahman al-Rahim (In the Name of God, the Merciful, the Compassionate).

Design and layout by Abir Usman

Published by
Great Books of the Islamic World, Inc.

Distributed by
KAZI Publications, Inc.
3023 W. Belmont Avenue
Chicago IL 60618
Tel: 773-267-7001; FAX: 773-267-7002
email: info@kazi.org

Contents

Endnotes

Introduction by Laleh Bakhtiar

In the Name of God, the Merciful, the Compassionate

I. Biographical Sketch

The "Prince of Physicians," Abu Al Sina (Avicenna) (b. 370/980) was born in Afshana, near Bukhara. By the age of ten he had learned the entire Quran as well as grammar and then began the study of logic and mathematics. Once these subjects were mastered, he studied physics, metaphysics and medicine. By the age of sixteen he had mastered all of the sciences of his day except metaphysics. While he had read Aristotle's Metaphysics over and over again and had even memorized it, he could not understand it until he read al-Farabi's commentary on it. Avicenna was then eighteen years old.

He was favored by the ruler of Bukhara because of his mastery of medicine, but when he was thirty-two, he was forced to migrate because of the political situation in his home town area. He migrated to Jurjan on the southeast coast of the Caspian Sea in an attempt to join the court of the well-known Qabus ibn Wushmgir. This never materialized as the ruler had died in 1013 during Avicenna's travels to Jurjan. Avicenna then retired to a village near Jurjan where he was to meet his disciple-to-be, al-Juzjani.

Al-Juzjani was devoted to Avicenna and was to write commentaries upon his works as well as to preserve copies of all of the master's writings. It was in Jurjan in 1012 that Avicenna wrote the beginning of his great medical text, *The Canon (al-Qanun)* on medicine. Avicenna remained in Jurjan for two or three years before moving to Rey in 405/1014 or 406/1015, a city near present day Tehran and from there to Hamadan in the northwest Iran. He became a minister in the Buyuid Court of Shams al-Dawlah as well as the court physician. Once again Avicenna was obliged to migrate because of the unstable political conditions in Hamadan so he moved to Isfahan where he enjoyed a fifteen year period of peace, writing many of his major works at that time.

Eventually, however, he was forced to migrate once again and moved back to Hamadan where he died in 428/1037.

II. Avicennian Corpus

One of the leading scholars on Avicenna and the editor of this series, Seyyed Hossein Nasr, has written the following:

> The writings of Avicenna, of which nearly 250 have survived, if we take all his short treatises and letters into account, range over nearly every subject known to the medieval world. These works are mostly in Arabic, but occasionally in Persian, as for example, the *Danish namah-i ala* (The Book of Science Dedicated to Ala al-Dawlah), which is the first philosophic work in modern Persian. Avicenna's Arabic style in his earlier works is rather difficult and uneven; and it was only during his long sojourn in Isfahan-when under the criticism of certain literary experts, he began to study Arabic literature intensely-that his style became polished and perfected. The works written later in life, especially the *Isharat wa'l tanbihat*, testify to this change.
>
> Aviennna's philosophical works include his Peripatetic masterpiece *al-Shifa* (The Book of the Remedy), the Latin *Sufficientia*, which is the longest encyclopedia of knowledge ever written by one man, his Najat (The Book of Deliverance), which is a summary of the *Shifa, Uyun al-hikmah* (Fountains of Wisdom), and his last and perhaps greatest masterpiece *Isharat wa 'l-tanbihat* (The Book of Directives and remarks). In addition he wrote a large number of treatises on logic, psychology, cosmology, and metaphysics. There are also the "esoteric" works pertaining to his "Oriental Philosophy" of which the *Risalah fi'l ishq* (Treatise on Love), the Trilogy *Hayy ibn Yaqan* (The Living Son of the Awake), *Risalat al-Tair* (Treatise of the Bird) and Salaman wa Absal, the last three chapters of the *Isharat*, and *Mantiq al-mashriqiyin* (The Logic of the Orientals), which is a part of a larger work now lost, are the most important.
>
> In the sciences, also, Avicenna composed many small treatises dealing with particular problems in physics, meteorology, and so on, as well as sections contained in the larger compendia, especially the *Shifa*, in which is found the most complete exposition of his views on zoology, botany, and geology, as well as psychology, which in Peripatetic philosophy—and contrary to the view of the later schools like the *Ishraqiyyun* is considered as a branch of physics or natural philosophy. As for medicine, Avicenna composed the famous *Qanun*, or *Canon*, which is perhaps the most influential single work in the history of medicine and is still taught in the East today, the *Urjuzah fi'l-tibb* (Poem on Medicine), containing the principles of Islamic medicine in rhyming verses easy to memorize, and a large number of treatises in both Arabic and Persian on various diseases and drugs.
>
> In addition to his philosophical and scientific works, Avicenna wrote several poems in Arabic and Persian of which *Qasidat al-ainiyah* (Ode on the Soul) is deservedly the most famous. Moreover, he wrote several religious works which include not only treatises on particular religious subjects, such as the meaning of fate and free will, but also commentaries upon several chapters of the Quran.

This latter category is particularly important because it was primarily in these commentaries that Avicenna sought to harmonize reason and revelation along lines already begun by *al-Kindi, al-Farabi* and the *Ikhwan al-safa*, continued after him by *Suhrawardi*, and finally brought to its fruition by *Mir Damad* and *Mulla Sadra*. These writings add an important dimension to the already multidimensional corpus of Avicenna's literary output and emphasize the richness of a collection of writings which range from observational and even experimental science to ontology, from mathematics to gnosis and metaphysics, and from logic to commentaries upon the Sacred Book.[1]

III. The Theory and Practice of Islamic Medicine

The traditional concept of medicine[2] differs profoundly from the view held in the modern world because in the traditional view, the spaces —meridians, channels—within the body and what flows through them are of more significance in causing illness than the shapes or organs, members themselves. That is, the emphasis is on that which flows through the channels as the "place" of the soul.

A clear parallel can be seen in traditional Islamic architecture where space is considered to be one of the most direct symbols of Being and it is primordial, all-pervading and, in Islamic cosmology, the locus of the Universal Soul. Space is also structured. Whether one is referring to the macrocosm or the microcosm, they each contain three divisions: body, soul and spirit.

Traditional man tends towards a mode of comprehension which provides a metaphysical interpretation of life, an interpretation that precedes and goes beyond all external perception. This mode of comprehension, or initial interpretation, affects all of man's perceptions because it begins by situating him in the universe. Initially this interpretation determines his awareness of cosmic space as an externalization of the macrocosmic creation which is analogous to his own microcosmic self. This traditional Hermetic concept forms part of the world view incorporated into the Islamic perspective, a view in which the universe is composed of a macrocosm and microcosm, each containing three great divisions: the body (*jism*), the soul (*nafs*) and the spirit (*ruh*).[3]

Depending on one's perspective, one is either drawn from the body through the soul to the Divine Spirit in the external world or from the body inward through the soul to the Hidden Treasure or Divine Spirit within.

Two interpretations of this concept arise which, although apparently different, are essentially the same. In the first, God as Manifest (*al-Zahir*), is the reality of universal externalization. From within the concentric circles of the macrocosm, there is an outward movement from the earth as

> corporeal manifestation through an all-pervading soul to the enveloping heavens, viewed as the seat of the Divine Spirit. In the second, complementary view of God as Hidden (*al-Batin*), there is an inward movement within the microcosm of man, beginning with his physical presence and moving towards his spiritual center, the Hidden Treasure. The two schemes correspond to each other, at the same time that one is the reverse of the other.[4]

In this structured space, the human being knows where he or she is. Direction is meaningful.

> It is only with reference to the heavens that the apparent indefiniteness of space can be given direction. In this way space acquires a qualitative aspect. The order of the spheres and the movements through the six directions of north, south, east, west, up and down constitute the primary coordinate system within which all creation is situated. All traditional sciences share this common frame of reference.[5]

The concept of place (*makan*) follows a meaningful direction or orientation. A sense of place consists of both a container (*jism*, body) and the contained (soul, spirit, breath).

> [The concept of place] does not have a tangible existence, but exists in the consciousness of the beholder who visually perceives physical boundaries while his intellect perceives [the soul] and spirit as 'contained,' defined within the boundaries.[6]

Within this structured, oriented concept of space as the place of the soul, all of creation contains both active and passive possibilities. The idea of time in motion arises from the active aspect of space while seen in its passive aspect, it is manifested in matter or form which is directly a product of this movement. This concept—that the soul (space) and not the body (shape) should lead in the healing art—is central to an understanding of traditional medicine.

> The esoteric theory of causation describes this motion as the movement of the soul towards the Divine Spirit through space. Thus the locus of time and form is space, which simultaneously manifests its active and passive aspects through motion.[7]

This perspective is the basis for traditional medicine which looks for the simultaneous movement systems which create a continuous flow based on number—three main faculties, three major organs, three souls, four elements, four humours, nine temperaments, and which interact in space, the place of the soul, with the organs, tissues, membranes, etc.

Finally, we come to the concept of rhythm in time which is best described in terms of traditional music based upon the poem with which Jalal al-Din Rum begins his masterful *Mathnawi*.

Hearken to this Reed forlorn,
Breathing, even since twas torn
From its rushy bed, a strain
Of impassioned love and pain.

The Secret of my song, though near,
None can see and none can hear.
Oh, for a friend to know the sign
And mingle all his soul with mine!

'Tis the flame of Love that fired me.
'Tis the wine of Love inspired me.
Wouldst thou learn how lovers bleed.
Hearken, hearken to the Reed![8]

The continuity and harmony of music is well appreciated and may serve to elucidate another aspect of the spiritual meaning of time-form continuity. The reed, in Jalal al-Din Rumi's poem, contains the bifold characteristics of place. Physically, the reed exhibits a *zahir* or external form which is passive to its hollow interior or *batin*, wherein lies the active spirit of the instrument. The music of the reed is symbolically seen as the externalization of an interior movement, just as musical tones work through wind instruments from the inside out. He who hears the music is aware of the inner space and the harmonious encounter of its motion with its outer shell. This interaction, in the traditional view, represents a spiritual synthesis which regards the reed's *zahir* as the body and its *batin* as the spirit, which, through the music of the soul, yearns to return to the reed bed from whence it was plucked, must as man yearns to return to the One from whom he was issued.[9]

The concept of motion associated with the creation of time and space is explored also by Ibn Arabi in his discourses on initial creation and the subsequent manifestations, viewed as the 'Breath of the Compassionate.' Here 'the universe is annihilated at every moment and re-created at the next without there being a temporal separation between the two phases. It returns back to the Divine Essence at every moment while in the phase of contraction and is re-manifested and externalized in that of expansion. . . Creation is renewed at every instant and its apparent 'horizontal' continuity is pierced by the 'Vertical Cause' which integrates every moment of existence into its transcendent Origin.'[10]

Because of the concentration of traditional Islamic medicine on what flows through the inner spaces, it becomes a dynamic system. That is, the whole is present and operative in each individual locus in which each individual locus knows, so to speak, its position in the whole, its relation to center. The dynamic qualities of the elements can be understood as manifestations of an orderly action of faculties (drives, energies, powers) within a given system. The elemental qualities of our body's system are part of a dynamic field and each elemental quality, as it presents itself, gives expression to the exact constellation of faculty that is present at the point at which the element is situated, a dynamic quality that permits the elemental qualities to become the conveyors of meaning; that makes temperaments out of the succession of elements.

Thus, we have introduced the traditional concepts of the soul and its place in space with the traditional components of space: structured (body, soul, spirit), oriented (six directions), sense of place (container/contained), positive space continuity (what flows through space creates shapes), time-form simultaneity (active as motion, passive as form), and rhythm in time (breath, pulse). Now let us turn to Avicenna. He begins *The Canon* with a definition of the science of medicine:

> Medicine (*tibb*) is the science by which we learn the various states of the human body in health and when not in health, and the means by which health is likely to be lost and, when lost, is likely to be restored back to health. In other words, it is the art whereby health is conserved and the art whereby it is restored after being lost.

Avicenna insists that the human body cannot be restored to health unless the causes of both health and disease are determined. In categorizing the causes, he uses Aristotle's system:

> Medicine deals with the states of health and disease in the human body. It is a truism of philosophy that a complete knowledge of a thing can only be obtained by elucidating its causes and antecedents, provided, of course, such causes exist. In medicine it is, therefore, necessary that causes of both health and disease should be determined.
>
> Sometimes these causes are obvious to the senses but at other times they may defy direct observation. In such circumstances, causes and antecedents have to be carefully inferred from the signs and symptoms of the disease. Hence, a description of the signs and symptoms of disease is also necessary for our purpose. It is a dictum of the exact sciences that knowledge of a thing is attained only through a knowledge of the causes and origins of the causes—assuming there to be causes and origins. Consequently our knowledge cannot be complete without an understanding both of symptoms and of the principles of being.

There are four causes—material, efficient, formal, and final. On the subject of health and disease, we have the following:

The Material Causes

The material (*maddi*) cause is the physical body which is the subject of health and disease. This may be immediate as the organs of body together with their vital energies and remote as the humours and remoter than these, the elements which are the basis both for structure and change (or dynamicity). Things which thus provide a basis (for health and disease) get so thoroughly altered and integrated that from an initial diversity there emerges a holistic unity with a specific structure (or the quantitative pattern of organization) and a specific type of temperament (the qualitative pattern).

The material cause, then is the physical body, as viewed from the traditional perspective. It consists of the organs, the breath, the humours and the elements. We begin with the elements as Avicenna does.

The Elements

The primary constituents of the human body in traditional medicine are called "the elements." They are the basic building blocks for the science of medicine.

The four elements—earth, air, fire, and water—are the simplest particles of all that is material. They are the simplest particles of our bodies. To each of them are joined two qualities. Earth is dry and cold; water, cold and moist; air, hot and moist; and fire is hot and dry. Earth is contrary to air and water to fire. Union is possible because water serves as a means between earth and air and air as a means between water and fire. The elements, like musical tones, possess an inclination not only to ascend and descend, but also to move in a circular direction. Each element is joined by one of its qualities to that which is below and by the other to that which is above it. Water to earth beneath by coldness and to air above by moisture; air to water beneath by moisture and to fire above by heat; fire to air beneath by heat and to earth toward which it declines by dryness; earth to water above by coldness and to fire which declines toward it by dryness. Two of the elemental qualities are active and two passive. Active are hot and cold. Passive are dry and wet. The resulting qualities, the ideal combination, is an equitable one.

Quality results from the opposing qualities of the elements, a mixture of hot, cold, wet and dry. Balance comes when the strength of primary qualities are equal to these qualities—an average of these qualities. In medicine, it does not depend upon exactly equal but "equitable," meaning that the quality and quantity of the elements are distributed in such a manner that the resulting pattern or equilibrium of the body as a whole or if its parts is the one most appropriate for that person.

When one quality predominates over the other, the body is not well suited to the needs of the soul. The proportion in which the elements are united with the body has an influence upon action. Slow and heavy moving signifies a predominance of cold and dryness (earth); fearfulness and sluggishness, of cold and wetness (water); cheerfulness, of heat and wetness (air); and sharp, angry violence, of heat and dryness (fire).

All physical forms consist of elemental qualities prefigured in the physical process. If something changes in the element, something must have changed in the physical process. The two stand to each other in the strict relationship of cause and effect.

As phenomena of the external world and, in traditional medicine, the inner world, consist of the elements and their qualities, as well. Different elemental qualities are always based on the different properties of the elements (higher, lower, lighter, heavier, colder, hotter, etc.). The distinguishing characteristic of the elements is that they differ like two colors, red and green, and like two shades of a single color, light and dark blue or like shapes rough and square. The property is a characteristic of such a nature that it both distinguishes different elements from one another and at the same time orders them in definite ways.

The dynamic quality of the elements is that they have direction. The elements point one to another—attract and are attracted—and are therefore directional forces. Elemental motion has its origin not in differences of properties but in differences of dynamic quality as conveyors of motion.

The Humours

The humours are the primary fluids of the body which move through inner space. These humours affect the function of the body and are themselves influenced by the states of motion and rest of the human being.

Food and drink are transformed into innate heat through the digestive process. The humours arise in the second stage of digestion in the liver. This process produces four humours which sustain and nourish the body and move through the channels or meridians: sanguineous (blood), serous (phlegm), bilious (choler, yellow bile) and atrabilious (melancholy, black bile) corresponding to air (hot and wet), water (cold and wet), fire (hot and dry) and earth (cold and dry). These are subject to variation in quantity and in degree of purity.

Illness results from either a quantitative or qualitative change of humour. In a "normal" state, the humours are assimilated by the organs and completely integrated into the tissues. In an "abnormal" state, due to improper digestion, the material is unsuitable for assimilation and therefore eliminated by the body. Surpluses may be eliminated by exercise, bathing, coition, purges and laxatives.

The sanguineous humour (blood), which is an equal temper, exceeds the others in proportion to quantity, is hot and moist, sweet and red. It imparts strength and color to the body and serves for the engendering of the drives. Located in the heart, it relates to Leo, Aries and Sagittarius in the Zodical constellations.

The serous humour or phlegm, next to blood in quantity, is watery, cold, moist and white. It moderates the strength, heat, and thickness of blood, nourishes the brain, and moistens and nourishes such part of the body as are concerned in motion. If blood fails, heat dissolves the serous humour into blood. Cancer, Pisces and Scorpio, as Zodiacal signs, relate to serous humour.

The bilious humour, least in quantity, is hot and dry, yellow or red and bitter. A part of it passes from the liver to the gallbladder and a part, flowing thence with other humours, moderates moisture and makes the blood subtle so that it may pass easily through straight ways. The bilious humour prevents the body from becoming heavy, sleepy and dull. It penetrates and opens passages and feeds members of the body in which the fiery element predominates. Zodiacal signs are Gemeni, Aquarius, and Libra.

The atrabilious humour is earthy and gross, thick, black and sour. A part of it passes to the spleen and a part remains with the blood. This humour feeds the bones, the spleen and other parts of the body which are gross or "melancholy" in nature. It tempers the two hot humours (sanguineous and bilious) and serves to stay and retain the floating spirits that arise from blood. The atrabilious humour thickens the blood and thus prevents it from flowing too freely through the veins and arteries. Within the Zodaic this humour is related to the three signs Tarus, Virgo, and Capricorn.

From the natural predominance of a humour in the human being spring definite characteristics of physique and conduct. Those dominated by the sanguinious humour are cheerful, courageous, kind and ingenious. Their blood, if subtle, makes the wit keen. As fatness increases, blood diminishes. The serous humour dominating is visible in people who are easily provoked, given to treachery and vehement in action; fierce in assailing but inconstant in sustaining the assault; inclined to envy, pride, prodigality and wrath. If the serous humour is corrupt, they are subject to evil passions and dreadful nightmares. Those with a predominance of bilious humour are generally slothful, given to bodily pleasures, sleepy, idle, dull of wit, heavy and slow. They love delicate food and drink. Those dominated by the atrabilious humour are hard to please, obstinate, suspicious, sorrowful and given to fearful thoughts.

The humours are exceedingly variable in quantity and quality. The sanguineous reigns from 3 am to 9 am; bilious from 9 am to 3 pm; serous from 3 pm to 9 pm and atrabilious from 9 pm to 3 am. The sanguineous humour increases in the spring. The heat of summer dissolves superfluities, wastes the humours and opens the pores. The breath escapes from the body with exhalations, moisture and vapors. The bilious humour is in ascendancy. Autumn breeds the serous humour.

Winter thickens the humours, constrains the sinews and sends natural heat inward. The atrabilious humour increases and makes people sluggish.

The active elemental qualities—cold and heat—form the humours. When heat is equable, the sanguineous humour forms; when heat is in excess, bilious humour forms; when in great excess so that oxidation occurs, atrabilious humour forms. When the cold is equable, serous humour forms; when cold is in excess so that congelation becomes dominant, atrabilious humour forms.

In addition to this, there are three souls within the human form:

> . . . namely, the vegetable, animal and rational, all of which descend from the world above and each of which possesses its own faculties. The more refined the mixture of the humours the greater the perfection and the more complete and perfect the possibility of receiving the soul. Moreover, in each man, health means the harmony of the humours and illness the disruption of the balance of the constitution. Of course the harmony is never perfect in any person, but relative to his own constitution, health means the re-establishment of the balance of the humours. Diagnosis for such disorders as fever are, in fact, based on searching for the way in which the balance of the humours has been upset. But for diseases which show overt signs, the most notable sign or signs are made use of it for diagnostic purposes and often the disease receives the name of the leading sign connected with it.[11]

Flowing in the space intermediate between the physical body and the force of life, is a placeless space, a space that, as a whole, has a direction and must have a center, the position toward which it is directed. Health or lack of it is is out from this center.

The Breath

The breath acts as the link between the body, soul and spirit. It is the breath which makes the perfect equilibrium of the elements possible.

God created the left side of the heart and made it hollow in order that it should serve both as a storehouse of the breath and as the seat of manufacture of the breath. He also created the breath to enable the drives of the "soul' to be conveyed into the corresponding members. In the first place the breath was to be the rallying-point for the faculties of the soul and in the second place it was to be an emanation into the various members and tissues of the body (whereby these could manifest the functions of those drives).

Now He produced the breath out of the finer particles of the humours and out of igneity and at the same time produced the tissues themselves (the visible body) out of the coarser and earthy particles of these humours. In other words, the breath is related to the attenuated particles as the body is related to the coarser particles of the same humours. Just as the humours are intermingled to produce a temperamental "form," whereby the members of the body are enabled to receive a physical appearance, impossible were they separate, so the attenuated portions of the humours, being intermingled into a temperamental form, enable the breath to receive the powers of the soul—impossible were the humours separate.

The beginning of the breath is as a divine emanation from potentiality to actuality proceeding without intermission or stint until the form (preparation, state) is completed and perfected. Each member, though derived from the self-same substance of the humours, nevertheless has its own particular temperament—for the proportional qualities of the (denser portions of the) humours and the form of their commixture are peculiar to each member. Similarly, although derived from the same attenuated portions of the humours, nevertheless each of the three breaths (natural, animal and vital) has its own particular temperament, because the proportional quantities of the more attenuated portions of the humours and the manner of their commixture are peculiar to each breath.

Although the body consists of several organs, there is one from which they all originally arose. As to what this organ actually was, there are various opinions. The fact remains that one organ necessarily came to light before other organs could arise out of it. Exactly the same is true in the case of the breaths. There is one single breath which accounts for the origin of the others. This breath, according to the most important philosophers, arises in the heart, passes thence into the principal centers of the body, lingering in them long enough to enable them to impart to it their respective temperamental properties. Lingering in the cerebrum it receives a temperament whereby it is capable of receiving the drives of sensation and movement; in the liver, it receives the drive of nutrition and growth (vegetative drives); in the generative glands it acquires a temperament which prepares it for receiving the drive of generation (reproduction).

The breath is similar to the spirit and is of three kinds:

(1) The vital spirit, hot and dry, has its center in the left ventricle of the heart, preserves life, causes the body to grow, move and reproduce, and travels through the arteries. (2) The psychic spirit, cold and wet, has its center in the brain, causes sensation and movement and moves through the nerves and is the source of movement and reason. (3) The natural spirit, hot and wet, has its center in the liver, is concerned with the reception of food, growth and reproduction and travels through the veins.[12]

Traditional medicine is first concerned with the rhythmic continuity of the breath itself and then the synthesis of breath as "time in motion" or "active space" and organs or members as "passive possibilities of space" of matter and form. Harmonic order brings together those two concepts of breath and organs which appear to be opposite but which inwardly contain one another and are therefore complements. The synthesis is achieved because the breath occupies a continuous space defined by passageways, meridians, channels which move through the shapes of organs, bones, muscles. Movement coalesces breath and organs into a unity.

The Organs

The humours in turn act as the constituent elements for the members or organs of the body which "are derived primarily from the commingling of the humours, just as the humours are derived primarily from the commingling of the aliments and the aliments are primarily composed of commingled elements. The organs are divided into simple ones having homogeneous parts such as flesh, bones, and nerves, and compound organs such as the hands and face. The organs are the instruments by which the passions and actions of the mind are achieved and act as its servants.

The primary elemental quality of an organ is based on its nutrient while its secondary quality is determined by what it excretes.

Hot organs consist of the vital force and heart, blood, liver, flesh, muscle, spleen, kidneys, breasts, testicles, muscular coats of arteries, veins, skin of palm (which is evenly balanced).

Cold organs consist of phlegm, hair, bones, cartilage, ligaments, serous membranes, nerves, spinal cord, brain, solid and liquid fats and skin.

Moist organs consist of phlegm, blood, sold and liquid fats, brain, spinal cord, breast, testicles, lungs, liver, spleen, kidneys, muscles, and skin.

Dry organs consist of hair, bones, cartilage, ligaments, tendons, membranes, arteries, veins, motor nerves, heart, sensory nerves, skin.

The Efficient Causes

> The efficient (*failiya*) causes are capable of either preventing or inducing change in the human body. They may be external to the person or internal. External causes are: age, sex, occupation, residence, and climate and other agents which effect the human body by contact whether contrary to nature or not. Internal causes are sleep and wakefulness, evacuation of secretions and excretions, the changes at different periods of life in occupation, habits and customs, ethnic group and nationality.

The efficient causes are clear and vary with each individual. Whereas the elements, humours, breath and organs as the material cause are all from nature, the efficient causes develop out of the nurturing process.

The Formal Causes

> The formal (*suriyah*) causes are three: temperaments (*mizajat*) (or the pattern of constitution as a whole) and the faculties or drives (*qawa*) which emerge from it and the structure (the quantitative patterns).

Temperament

Temperament arises from the elements and humours and it determines the way in which the soul functions. Each animal and each organ of the body has a temperament of its own.

> The Almighty Creator has bestowed upon every animal and every one of its organs the most appropriate and the best adapted temperament for its various functions and passive states.
>
> Since the verification of this truth is a matter for philosophers and not physicians, we may accept that the human being has been bestowed a most befitting temperament and most appropriate faculty or drives for the various active and passive states in the body. Similarly, every organ and member is endowed with the proper temperament appropriate to its own functional requirement. Some He has made more hot, others more cold, others more dry and others more moist.

The temperament is "equable" when the contrary qualities are in perfect equilibrium, and out of harmony or "inequable" when the temperament tends toward a particular quality. Therapeutics, then, are based on the allopathic principle of contraries. That is, "cold" diseases can be cured by "hot" remedies and vice versa.

Avicenna then explains this method further:

> It is worth remembering that when a medicine is referred to as being evenly balanced, it does not mean that its temperament is the same as of a human being, or that it is even similar to it, for it would then be like a human being. It merely means that such a medicine, after being acted upon by the innate heat [metabolized] fails to produce any material change in the normal state of the body, and that its pharmacological actions remain within the limits of normal human temperament. In other words, when this medicine is given to a normal person, it does not produce any appreciable change or imbalance in the body. When it is said that a drug is hot or cold, it does not mean that the physical quality of the drug is particularly hot or cold or that it is colder or hotter than the human body. If this were so there would follow the unwarranted inference mentioned above that an evenly constituted medicine is the one which has exactly the same temperament as the human body. It means just that such a medicine produces a greater amount of heat or cold than what was originally present in the body. A drug which, for example, is cold for the human being may be hot for the scorpion, or the medicine which is hot for the human being may be cold for the serpent. In fact it may also mean that the same medicine may be less hot for one person than for another. This is the reason why physicians are advised to change their medicine when it fails to produce the desired result.

The growth and decay of the human body is dependent upon the human temperament. Growth depends upon the heat contained in the sperm which is gradually used up. Meanwhile, the moisture lessens in quantity and quality, thus preserving the innate heat at a constant level up to the old age. Ultimately, however, the moisture of the body comes to an end, and the innate heat i.e. extinguished, thus causing the death to which everyone is destined and which depends upon the original temperament of the human body.

The correspondences between the various orders of reality and the temperament have been summed up in the following:

> The uniqueness of the temperament of each individual indicates that each microcosm is a world of its own, not identical with any other microcosm. Yet, the repetition of the same basic humours in each constitution bears out the fact that each microcosm presents a morphological resemblance to other microcosms. Moreover, there is an analogy between the human body and the cosmic order, as shown by the correspondence between the humours and elements. There is in the Hermetico-alchemical natural philosophy, which was always closely tied

to medicine in Islam, a basic doctrine of the correspondence between all the various orders of reality: the intelligible hierarchy, the heavenly bodies, the order of numbers, the parts of the body, the letters of the alphabet which are the "elements" of the Sacred Book, etc. The seven cervical and the twelve dorsal vertebrae correspond to the seven planets and the twelve signs of the Zodiac, as well as to the days of the week and the months of the year; and the total number of discs of the vertebrae, which they consider to be twenty-eight, to the letters of the Arabic alphabet and the stations of the moon. There is, therefore, both numerical and astrological symbolism connected with medicine, although the closeness of the relation has not been the same during all periods of Islamic history, nor among all the medical authorities. But the correspondence and "sympathy" (in the original sense of the word "sympathia") between various orders of cosmic reality form the philosophical background of Islamic medicine.[13]

The Faculties or Drives

The body also possesses faculties which originate the functions of various organs. The major faculties are (1) the vital (*hayawaniyah*), responsible for preserving the integrity of the breath, sensation, and movement of the heart; (2) the natural (*tabiiyah*) governing the nutritive powers of the liver and the reproductive powers of the generating organs; and (3) the animal (*nafsaniyah*) controlling the brain and the rational faculty.

The powers of the various members are due to the vital faculty[14] which provides the body with its inner force. The vital faculty is that which appears in the breath at the very moment at which the breath develops out of the rarefied particles of the humours.

Between the human body as a whole and the individual points as its parts there is a relationship—the whole being given with and active in the part and the part being aware that it is part and directly announcing its relation to the whole. Whenever we encounter a phenomenon showing this relationship between whole and parts we may assume, that a force, an ordered action of forces, is the basis. This is the role of the faculties which we can only know through their effects. They work through the physical body without ever touching it.

The Final Causes

The final (*tamamia*) causes are the actions or functions. They can be understood only from a knowledge of both the faculties or drives (*qawa*) and the vital energies (breaths, *arwah*) that are ultimately responsible for them. These will be described presently.

IV. Conclusion

The power of traditional Islamic medicine is in realizing that space leads and forms shapes; shapes then interact with space and space with the breath/inner light with which every human being has been endowed. What he or she does with that determines the extent of their completion and perfection.

O. Cameron Gruner's Remarks

During the past fifty years,[1] the popular imagination has been stirred by a succession of important discoveries in the domain of medicine and surgery. The triumphs of the latter field have been spectacular to a degree. Those of medicine have been much less conspicuous, chiefly because the mind must inquire into them before it can properly appreciate them. How much does not humanity owe to the steadily continued researches in bacteriology, and the painstaking observations which have revealed the life-cycles of many of the parasites to which tropical and other diseases are due and to the whole procedure of immuno-therapy, the just pride of scientific as distinct from clinical medicine, and the outcome of all these researches?

As compared with all this, the speculative subtleties of former times appear both futile and unworthy of resuscitation. But the ancient system was not as valueless as is so generally supposed. Taking as an adequate criterion the first book of *The Canon of Medicine* of Avicenna, which is here presented [almost in its entirety], and is fairly representative of the whole work, we find in its pages references to many departments of human knowledge—(though it might be objected that all these departments of knowledge are now separate sciences, each requiring its own professorial staff, its own literature, and journals and that they are not mentioned under the special names with which we are familiar, their existence in those days cannot be denied) cosmology, anatomy, physiology, and psychology; the: various branches of clinical medicine-etiology, semiology, diagnosis, and prognosis; the departments of therapeutics-hygiene, dietetics, balneology, and climatology, in addition to materia medica, pharmacology, and pharmacy. Moreover, the reader is presumed to be conversant with logic, criteriology, and metaphysics.

The presence of obvious literal errors in the work must not lead us to commit the more serious mistake of overlooking the fact that it is entirely built up upon a sound philosophy of human nature, which is as vitally important today, though largely ignored in former times. The traditional medicine was concerned essentially with the given patient now before us; whereas now it is simply the science of diseases which it is our duty to diagnose accurately, prevent if possible, and treat on lines capable of wholesale application. To Avicenna, the determination of the constitution of the patient was of the very first importance, because on it depended the character, course, and duration of his illness, and upon that again depended the choice of remedies.

After all, from the patient's point of view, the real object of consulting a medical man is to be restored to a state of well-being. It is little comfort to be virtually told that 85-90 percent of cases of his complaint are cured by the treatment adopted in his case, only to find that he proves to be one of the remaining 10-15 percent for whom there is little or nothing to be done. True, his sighs are drowned in the shouts of the fortunate, and fail to reach the clinical laboratory, surgical wards, consulting room or research councils.

If, in the interests of these few, chance leads us to the pages of this traditional work, it would seem that suggestions occur in it which enable us to understand their plight, and thereby help them to understand it also. Even if the enemy is not put out of action, his enmity is less evident when he is understood.

It has been the aim of this treatise to elaborate Avicenna's central theme by references to the various philosophies extant in his time—Sufi, Vedantic, Buddhist, Chinese; to Persian writings subsequent to his time (Rumi, Sadi, Shabistari, etc.); and to views presented by various modern philosophies, including western theosophy.

But these various directions of thoughts are not drawn upon in order to elaborate a composite system after the fashion of theosophical eclecticism. On the contrary, readers accustomed to various modes of thought are invited across a bridge leading from their various starting-points, across the chasm of modernism, until they reach the concise teaching of Thomistic philosophy, wherein all other aspects of the one truth receive their proportionate places. The inclusion of ideas from writers whose ideas appear to be altogether of the by-ways may torment a few, but may also help a few to see the: greater thing, and thereafter be content to stay upon the broad highway to which the several paths have converged.

Science has been removed from its usual role of master, and has been pressed into service, and that service is to illuminate the subject of human nature. To quote a recent paper,[2] "Under the great swelling flood that represents the growing complexity of modern medicine, let us not allow ourselves hold fast to that great life-saving conception of the essential unity of the human body. Let us oppose fearlessly those currents of medical thought that tend to isolate—arbitrarily and to the detriment of true knowledge—the various segments of this one great subject. Let us welcome all methods, all discoveries, that help the one man in charge of the one patient to broaden the base of his attack, to widen the sweep of his beneficent vision." These words were possibly expressed with a different object, but apply well to the theme of this treatise.

The old teaching about "constitution" should undergo a mutual intergrowth with the knowledge of modern science, pervaded throughout with the fundamental teaching of Thomistic philosophy, when there would emerge the beginnings of a possible system of modern scholastic medicine—thoroughly logical, plain, free of mystery, free of materialism, but not ignoring the so-called "occult" and metaphysical; with the knowledge of the nature of the constitution of the individual patient as its central and dominant theme. Were the whole medical training along such lines, the student would be able to approach his clinical instruction thoroughly aware that the individuality of the patient comes first, and that the ailment from which he suffers is but part and parcel of one single story, and not merely an accidental superposition. But the student would constantly need guidance to ensure his over-riding the disregard or ignorance, if not actual rejection, of scholastic principles which characterizes the concrete modern teaching of pathology in its various departments.

The following brief survey of the most important teachings of *The Canon.*

Teachings of The Canon

The General Notion of the Nature of a Human Being

The following three propositions belong to it: (1) the human being (MF)[3] is composed of matter and a principle of life, the two together making him "he" or "she," he or she is "a single substance endowed with a natural tendency to realize and maintain the conditions of its organization." (2) This principle of life comprises three main groups of potential and actual activities—the vegetative, the sensitive and the rational. This multi-potentiality of the principle of life is represented in the expression "bundle of life." (3) The organs of the body are the material manifestations (the actualities) of the several potentialities The vegetative organs belong to the "vegetative soul," the sense-organs and appurtenances belong to the "sensitive soul." The intelligence and will belong to the "rational soul," which has not literal organs but acts through the instrumentation of the organs of the vegetative and sensitive systems. All these components belong intimately together apart from macroscopic or microscopic boundaries it.

These propositions are further defined by the following negative statements: (1) the human being is not a collection of molecules and forces; he manifests chemical, electric, and other phenomena, which are not causes, but effects. (2) The organs are not distinct from the powers they exhibit. (3) The brain is not the producer of thought.

The remarkable action which the human being achieves by his complicated mechanical contrivances are distinct from himself, whereas in the human being the mechanism and the manipulator are the self same. Even when there is as grave mechanical interference with organs as occurs in hemiplegia, or in the cortical lesions of insanity, the rational soul remains untouched, though no longer able to communicate its activities to the outer world. To quote from St. Thomas, "The intellect, being a power that does not make use of a corporeal organ, would in no way be hindered in its act through the lesion of a corporeal organ, if for its act there were not required the act of some power that does make used of a corporeal organ."[4]

Thought is produced by the activity of the rational souls; the changes in the brain—whether chemical, cytological, or otherwise—are not causes, but the visible effects of the activity. (4) There is no bridge over the gulf between rational life and the-vegetative sensitive life; the distinctions are radical. (5) The life-principle is not subject to the laws of inheritance, those which govern matter; it is not divisible into organs, or parts, or elements. As soon as it ceases to operate, it is left behind the material body, which though apparently the same is actually quite different from the animate person recently before me.

The Notion of the Constitution of Any Given Individual When in Health

This notion should be made as tangible as possible.[5] The constitution may be expressed in terms of a number of formula to be taken together—a series of "notes," some of which are constants, and others variables. In this formula, the qualities are represented by the initials of their corresponding names; the quantities are represented by index numbers from 1 to 5, to stand for slight, moderate, normal, marked, and very marked, and very marked respectively.

The Constants

I. *The Body:* (1) general physique [good, poor, robust, spare, strong, delicate]; (2) dominant "element" [example: $E^2W^2F^5A^3$] for earth, water, fire and air; (3) dominant "humour," shown in the humoural formula [example: $S^3L^1B^5A^8$] for sanguineous, serous (lymphatic), bilious, and atrabilious]. This formula is really descriptive of the "temperament," but the latter word bears a different meaning in modern popular usage. (4) The absolute or relative strength or weakness (functional capacity) of the several organs; hypo, hyper-function. [example: $V^4T^4M^2O^3N^1G^3$, for vegetative (i.e. alimentary), thoracic (i.e. respiratory and circulatory), muscular (including skeletal), osseous (including genito-urinary), nervous (including sympathetic system) and glandular (including haemopoietic, endocrine, and hepatic) types. (5) The emotional make-up, or formula [example: $G^3L^2T^1I^5$ (gaudium, laetitia, timor, ira),[6] from which the dominant passion and its modifiers are noted. The modern use of the word "temperament" belongs here.

The difference in capacity is partly explained by considering the time-factor,[7] and partly as a fundamental difference.[8] All the material brought to an organ, whether nutritive, or excretory, is not at once taken up in its entirety; only a certain proportion is removed and the remainder passes on, so that the blood has its composition at a certain level. The modern threshold values recognize this fact. The time-factor is of very great importance.

II. *The Mind:* here comes the description of the disposition, the type of mind, or mental make-up.[9] Mental capacity may be expressed in terms of the relative or absolute strength or weakness of the various faculties, enumerated under "talents" (which are simply developments of particular faculties above the average).[10]

> "The better the disposition of a body, the better the soul allotted to it which clearly appears in things of different species: and the reason thereof is that act and form are received into matter according to matter's capacity thus because some men have bodies of better disposition, their souls have a greater power of understanding . . . . This occurs in regard to the lower powers of which the intellect has need in its operation, because those in whom the imaginative, cogitative and memorative powers are of better disposition, are better disposed to understand."[11]

The mental attitude towards things, which emerges from the character, is also to be noted, for sometimes this may explain the cause of the illness (i.e., wanton exposure to infections in spite of warnings), and will show whether the patient is suppressing relevant facts, will respond to treatment, or is secretly concerned with some fear or doubt which is the real object of his visit to the doctor. Moreover, knowledge of this aspect of character will safeguard the physician himself, either by making him aware of the patient's possible cynical opinion about a profession he is unfortunately obliged to deal with, or, more important, by enabling him to avoid offering advice which is palpably foolish to an intelligent patient.

The Variables

The degree of vitality: this is also spoken of as the strength of innate heat in the text;[12] (2) deviations from the functional capacities normal to the individual; (3) the nature or degree of "resistance." In terms of *The Canon*, this would be expressed in the "humoural formula," and in terms of "obstructions" of various kinds. These account for the "soil" which renders declared disease: (a) possible; or (b) amenable to alteration by artificial means.[13]

Foreign though such data are to modern clinical work, they are often actually employed in ordinary conversation, as when one describes a person as sanguine, or bilious, or phlegmatic, or as of saturnine temperament. Some adjective descriptive of the emotional make-up is not infrequent in case reports degrees of vitality are spoken of seriously by the laity, diplomatically by the practitioner.

In so far as they provide a simple means of codifying tentative knowledge upon complex and elusive individual characteristics which it is our duty to notice, the data are all worth consideration.

The Notion of the Nature of the State of Disease

The vegetative processes associated with digestion and absorption of food may be first briefly referred to. The picture of the whole nutritive cycle is comprehended in the idea of the "liver."[14] We trace the food constituents through the columnar cells of the intestinal mucosa, across the areolar tissue into the vascular roots of the portal and lacteal system; then into the liver unit itself (comprising phagocytic secretary cells, fundal cells, cubical excretory cells, and the hepatic arterioles and lymphatic clefts related to the sinusoids); then into the general blood-stream, and finally out of the body through various organs, including the goblet cells of the intestinal mucosa, the bile-ducts, the pancreas, etc. The extra-hepatic portion of the cycle is nearly co-terminous with the rest of the body.

To complete this picture we first remember the relation between the quality of food and the quality of chyme; then we consider how the ultimate components of the food travel (N-compounds, glucose, fat, phosphorus, sulphur, iron, and the like)—during rest, exercise, sleep, etc. and according to the character of the diet as a whole, the fluids taken, and the state of the bowels, etc. We may realize that they are manifested in the blood in the form of alkaline tide, viscosity, fibrin-content, and the various morphological changes revealed by blood-examination. We picture also the innumerable chemical interchanges and physical transformations in various parts of the cycle; the formation of waste-substances, and the factors on which the whole of the processes depend. [15] In brief, then our picture of the body is that of a complex of tubes and channels —potential as well as actual—which vary in size from the obvious alimentary-canal, air-passages, and great blood vessels, down to the finest ramifications of the latter, the cavernous tissues—both macroscopic and microscopic—the serous cavities, and the intracellular channels. All these form one continuous labyrinthine system, through which we may trace the ingested food materials, the metabolic, secretory and excretory products. As long as these channels are patent throughout, and As long as these various subs stances (including the "breath of life") can flow freely through them, and the vital energy has a free play outward, so long is the body in a state of health.

But as soon as there is a continued interference with the freedom of movement, even though it be merely an ebb and flow that is affected, in any part of the canalicular system, then a state of disease arises, culminating in histological anatomical changes. Hence, when we observe a case of illness, we may be sure there is some "obstruction" in some channels in some part of the body—not necessarily in that where the symptoms occur (i.e., the nasal discharge of "cold in the head," the bronchial expectoration in bronchitis, the serous effusion into the pleura, the respiratory phenomena in an attack of asthma, are manifestations in the respiratory system of obstructions elsewhere).

The next addition to the picture of the sick person's state is furnished by the causes of the obstruction. Avicenna considered these under two groups, the '"material" (i.e. those in which "matter" is concerned) or "humoural diseases" and the non-material. To the latter group would belong cases of gross obstruction, such as by compression from without, or such as by obstruction with calculi and those in which there is a functional disorder—hypo-function, hyper-function, dysfunction. For instance, in renal disease, the loss of functional capacity may render the-normal ebb and flow of substances disorderly.[16]

The group of humoural diseases is predominant in Avicenna's pathology, and if we bear in mind what the "humours" really are, this position becomes quite reasonable. Perverted metabolism is associated with changes of physical state in the fluids of the body. Limpid fluids may become viscid, viscous substances may become mobile or "tenuous." In the ancient work, these chemical changes were thought of, not in "equations," but under interchanges between the imponderable elements, as being subject to the laws of *uruj, nasul, jalal, jamal, qada, qadr*,[17] the rhythm, phases and rate of movement of the "breath" and the fluctuations of degrees of innate heat. Concrete examples are such as: precipitation of urates in tissues, altered reaction of tissue juices in rheumatoid arthritis, cardio-renal disease, tuberculosis; variations of content of Ca, Na, Mg, etc., in the tissue-water, so that the flow from tissue to blood and vice versa is impeded.[18]

The Canon often insists on the presence of "superfluities" as a cause of "obstructions" of the canalicular system not only in the tangible four humours, but also in regard to the "breath."[19] In the latter case, the substance of the breath (i.e. water-vapor) ceases to be "bright," and "clear," and its odor becomes offensive, and its freedom of flow is impaired .

Finally, adding from modern knowledge, there are the changes in the fluids of the body produced by bacterial or putrefactive breakdown—whether this begins in intestinal stasis or arises in the course of specific bacterial infections. There are then obstructions not only in the old sense, but in the form of the successive histological lesions consequent—vascular, nutritional, and inflammatory. Materials are deposited more or less permanently (irreversible reactions), as i.e., solid odema, collagenous tissue, scar formation, fibrosis, and hyalo-fibrosis, adipose tissue, hyperplastic formations. Loss of anatomical patency is super added to loss of functional perviousness.

Clearly, whereas we give first place to the bacterial invasion, Avicenna gave it to the habits of life. He was deeply impressed by the obvious fact that the quality of food determines the kind of chyme, and that the kind of chyme determines the quality of the freedom of flow through the diffuse canalicular system of the body. As they accumulate in the stagnating tissue-juices they come to exercise a noxious action; they come to be beyond the capacity of the third and fourth digestions (tissue-digestion), and with their stagnation, the ever-circulating bacteria (taken up with the food) also settle and multiply and wandering-cell infiltrations gather together. The beginnings of disease are laid down. The functional disturbance has been succeeded by anatomical lesions.[20]

Finally, Avicenna enlarges his view of humoural disease by noting the influence of many extracorporeal factors[21] as well as the period of life, not to mention "the decree of God."[22] Thus, one and the same kind of food taken at the "warm" period of life in the "warm" season may contribute more to the formation of a given humour than at another.

If we knew the patient's formula, and how the climactic and other conditions are likely to affect it, and whether they are compatible or not with susceptibility to the agents at work, our composite picture of the patient's state would be of great value, and illnesses often inexplicable would lose their mystery. How much more efficient might not the treatment be, if the remedial measures in contemplation were selected to harmonize with them?

No doubt only a fanatic would note the barometer, thermometer, humidity, hours of sunshine, wind-direction and velocity, the character of previous seasons, the clues afforded by then migration so insects, rodents, and birds, the presence or prevalence of certain parasites in a district, and the many other points noted in Part Three[23] before prescribing the regimen for the patient. But it would seem that some Eastern physicians of bygone times conscientiously strove to learn from such factors.

The Guides to the Diagnosis of the State of the Patient

The patient before us is as a manuscript written in some highly complex language which it is our business to decipher. The alphabet is furnished by the several colors, the simple observations of size, shape, consistency, contour, texture, and the like. The vocabulary consists of the external features both in repose and animation, and of the physical signs as taught to-day. The grammar lies in the "general guides" (sphygmology, urinoscopy, examination of feces and blood). The language is to be translated into: states of natural (vegetative), sensitive, and emotional instinctive drives, functional capacities, plethora, obstructions, solutions of continuity, etc. that is, the state of the whole composite, in all aspects. This task can only be accomplished imperfectly at the best, even by the most skilled and most learned. Our silent teachers, or guides, the "indications" always enable us to ascertain something, and we must perforce be content with that on the present occasion and be determined to use this experience as the guide to better success on the next.

One of the guides suggested in *The Canon* lies in one's own state of health. Properly to interpret what we observe, we must ourselves have no disharmony of functions arising from errors of diet, no deposit in the urine, no weight in the bowels, no obstructions in our own brain, no mental fatigue, no emotional pre-occupation, no rigid notions regarding etiology or prognosis; there must be clear channels for the breath, and the breath must be under the control of the will. It must be kept pure by recollection, by devotion, and observance of prayer. The reason for this is that under such conditions, long persevered, we are enabled to receive an "impression" from the patient. We become aware of his atmosphere, aura, or personality in the form of an idea of his degree and kind of vitality. But unless this impression is registered rapidly, namely at the first approach of the patient, it will be confused and illegible by reason of the mutual inter-impression of one's own vitality with his. In another idiom, we observe "with the eye of a Taoist." In our own idiom, we make use of sound reasoning power, common sense, and a certain kind of "intuition," or "clinical sense."

The guides furnished by general observation of the patient are, in brief: (1) external features in repose: (a) colors of face, hair, skin, eye (sclerae, iris); (b) odors and savors; (c) form of the body: (i) as a whole; (ii) in detail. The features, the hands, the limbs; the relative proportions (length, breadth, and thickness) of nose, cheeks, upper lip, lower lip, chin, mouth, ears, orbit, eyebrows, forehead, etc.; the character of the neck, shoulders, etc. (2) Features when animated: (a) expression, gaze, look, facial gestures (vivacity, sleepiness, languidness); (b) deportment or attitude,24 gestures, carriage, specific acts or mannerisms, definitely morbid movements or defective movements. (c) voice: tone of voice, manner of speech (clear, loud, or the opposite); clues to the physical and mental type, and the degree of energy and vitality.

Space does not allow of any attempt to furnish precise details of the external signs of functional capacity of internal organs. The principle is exemplified thus: the lower part of the nose is part of the respiratory system, and shares in the degree of development of the whole system; therefore wide nostrils with well-formed aloe go with good development of the whole respiratory function, whereas narrow delicate nostrils and small alae refer the observer to some other system as well-developed. Large mouth, thick lips, large masseters, and generally well-developed lower part of the face go with good development of the digestive tract throughout. Moreover, development or capacity above the average in one system denotes relative weakness and functional deficiency in another system. The subject is extensive.[25]

Our general guides differs noticeably, from that revealed in *The Canon*. To follow Avicenna, (1) when one places the hand on the pulse, one absorbs oneself in it, without the distraction of a watch, until one has found out how it runs minute after minute. Even if it misses, without an intermission of the heart, because the patient gives a twitch of the finger or begins to talk, one learns even from that. The study of the circulation is more than the study of the heart's action. (2) When one examines the urine, even with all the apparatus of modern chemistry, we must remember that it is first and foremost the guide to the state of digestion—especially its "second stage" (that in the liver) as well as in the "third" stage (that in the small vessels). We are misled by the search for albuminuria and glycosuria, for many would make these abnormalities into diseases. Thus, the number of persons in whom albuminuria is not evidence of renal disease far outnumber those in which it is; the presence of such a substance in the urine should lead to the questions: is some substance not being dealt with? If so, why? Can only the kidney handle it? To follow a useful rule, the real trouble is remote. It may lie in the brain, in the emotional state (cf. Graves' disease, i.e., pentosuria, cystinuria, alkaptonuria also break the current ideas about urinalysis.[26] (3) As regards the guide furnished by the feces matter, again, our knowledge is much greater than was Avicenna's and we do not apply it in his terms. We are apt to lose ourselves in fat analyses, nitrogen estimations, occult blood tests, B. coli classifications. Negative results in each case are taken to mean nothing of note, regardless of the continual secretory and excretory changes proceeding in the intestinal mucosa, and the vitality of nerve-ganglia, etc. Essential and definite derangements may occur without conspicuous deviations from the restricted standards usually laid down.

The guide furnished by an examination of the brood may be spoken of as the most notable modern addition to Avicenna's three general guides. The data obtained from it—physical, physicochemical, cytological, serological—are very numerous, but are lost more often than not by restriction to the diagnosis of the various "blood-diseases." When properly applied, all the data obtained from the blood inform us of the functional state of all the organs and of the existence of the main groups of pathological state.[27]

Treatment

"The healing art, as it is described in books, is far inferior to the practical experience of a skillful and thoughtful physician." (Rhazes).

"Many are healed by the action of nature without the art of medicine."[28] "Man teaches by outward ministration, but God by inward operation: even so the physician is said to minister, to nature when he heals."[29]

Application of the principles of *The Canon* to modern practice would seem superfluous. The common ailments, especially those of minor surgery, are nowadays treated in stereotyped fashion, which appears to be beyond improvement. It is not with such cases that reference to *The Canon* is suggested. It is the general principle which may be reviewed in the mind, and lines of treatment such as were once in vogue may be quite usefully applicable in a few cases which do not well respond to modern methods. Moreover, the conscience of even the most careful may not be altogether clear in regard to the immemorial rule: "*tutto, cito, et jucunde*."

The subject may be briefly considered under two headings: plan of treatment; methods of treatment.

The Plan of Treatment

The choice of a plan of treatment depends on the view which is taken as to the cause of the illness. It is no new or modern thing to say "treat the cause." The distinction between new and old is in regard to the idea of the nature of the cause. In these days nearly every illness is ultimately due to an infection or intoxication, and the aim of treatment is to destroy the one and render the other innocuous. To Avicenna, illness was primarily an abnormal state of condition, to which many factors contributed. The scheme of treatment must, therefore, envisage them all. To facilitate this, the practitioner of those days would advisedly mentally review the whole of the second part.[30]

Indeed, if we scrutinize the subject more closely, it will appear that Avicenna's plan is after all very proper. For, even if we could attack the microbic cause specifically, there would still remain the lesions which it has produced, and the lowering of the vitality (=interferences with the flow of vital currents, in Paracelsus' idiom)[31] A condition remains to be combated; the condition is uppermost as far as the patient is concerned. Even in those relatively few cases in which the disease is bound up-with a particular organ, so that the name of the disease is according (i.e., gastric ulcer, cerebral hemorrhage), it is the condition we have to face. The cause, even when known, has done its work, and gone.

It is true that many other interpretations of disease and corresponding plans of treatment are put forward in various quarters from time to time, especially by the intellectually anarchistic. This occurrence is partly the outcome of the arbitrary attitudes towards patient and friends sometimes exhibited by some of the representatives of academic medicine and would be best met by frank and courteous enquiry into lay opinions. Not everyone subscribes to the restrictions of medical ethics, and the patient is too often treated as if illness ipso facto at once deprives him of ordinary intelligence. After all, he seeks medical help for a distinct object, and remuneration for the services is presumed, so that he is entitled to go elsewhere, at his own choice, if unfortunately in his particular case the plan and method of treatment proves unsuccessful. But this view is not subscribed to by those who assume that the whole of the knowledge needed for every case is comprehended within the orthodox teaching of the day, and that every individual possesses.

The Methods of Treatment

Even the methods of treatment set forth in The Canon are still resorted to at times. No doubt, we would do well to follow them more frequently. Thus, systematic purgation is often called for, but not carried out as radically as of old. Cupping is still of value for such conditions as lumbar myositis, acute hemorrhagic nephritis, and those diseases amenable to autohaemolysins. Venesection is sometimes effectively applied for cases of high blood-pressure, threatened apoplexy; it is incidentally used in the course of obtaining blood-tests.

Drug Treatment

The steady decline of drug treatment in modern medical practice is evidenced in several directions: (1) the steady removal, in successive editions of the *British Pharmacopceia* of herbal remedies which are supposed to have no action because laboratory animals appear to be unaffected by them; (2) the infrequency with which medicines are ordered for hospital patients; (3) the penalization of panel practitioners for "over-prescribing"; (4) the desire on the part of many lay persons to banish "drugs" as being "unnatural."

Inconsistencies are frequent. There is the strange perversity which (through legislation) denies facilities for the use of the few drugs whose potency is quite unquestionable. There is the subterfuge of resorting to placebos (which often cost no more than the bottle containing them). Those among the lay who decry drugs are pleased to employ herbal remedies. Where there is a popular demand for the latest remedies, this is met by a never-ending stream of new synthetic and other preparations, and costly manufactured products, which also the medical world submits to. Truly the mind ever seeks in the relatively inaccessible, and the expensive, that which lies all the time, and without price, at our feet. It describes as progress that which better knowledge would render superfluous.

The truth is that we know far too little about the herbal remedies of *The Canon*. To begin with we forget that they cannot be efficient without careful attention to the conditions of their cultivation (soil, climate, season, etc.), the times proper for their collections, the details of their preservations and the laws governing the formation and circulation of the active principles during the life-cycles of the various plants. We do not individually know how to identify adulterations, whether accidental or deliberate. We leave to wholesale manufacture that which was once properly undertaken individually since personal artistic skill may be the real condition for pharmacological efficiency. We adopt the short cut of standardization of drugs as the remedy for the loss of potency inevitable after neglect of such various factors. But even if the purity and potency of remedies be granted, by recourse to the best sources they must be employed with deliberate care.

As Avicenna shows in the second book of *The Canon*, there must be a knowledge of the constitution or individuality of the plants which yield the drug; harmony with the constitution of the patient must be aimed at. Out of a number of drugs of like action, some will accord better with one person as constitution than with another's. One remedy may soothe and ease without its specific action being at all diminished whereas another performs its work harshly and unpleasantly; another may be overpowered by the personal factor. The scope of the subject is great and its study with intent to serious practical application, should not require an apologia.

Such considerations as these open the door of romance. The discovery that all nature is a living whole, always at work, earnestly, steadily, continuously developing an fidea, would arouse a new and intensely absorbing interest—that of watching the unseen worker, though His hands are not to be discerned, that which He does is ever proceeding before us as a continual motion-picture, and we may become aware not only of the merely superficial fact of the movements, but also of the purpose unfolding.

Watching the medicinal trees and shrubs and herbs in this way, and seeing their properties by their forms, and colors and odors, and their changes in character with the changes of the seasons, and alternations of drought and plenty (variations of rate of growth, of activity of flowering and fruiting), how great is the wonder of the work of nature! We note how substances are being elaborated into plants which we, wanting their help, know how to take at the crucial moment—now we must draw the resin; now we must take these flowering tops, and so on. But we are not the only watchers. The bees have been waiting, the birds, the slugs, the ants, the herbivora all these and many others wait to draw from such supplies that which is applicable to their several requirements. Nature itself also waits for all these things to be collected from its treasury. Everything has been worked out; the interactions are arranged for they all belong to the purpose of the Designer; and He Himself is waiting for that over which He incessantly broods, with entire and complete intention. He too waits to draw out of Creation that which was His object in making it.

No doubt it is true that few of the ancient physicians entered fully into this inner life of the world of which they formed a part. Few even of those who learned *The Canon* by heart may have applied it effectively at all times and on all occasions; few may have meditated sufficiently to consider the soul-life of the patient they were called upon to help. But the life was there then, as it is here now. It could be read then, as it should be now. The entry to the infinite treasure-house of nature was not locked then, and it is not locked now. Indeed, the entry was not merely through one door, there was a portal of entry on every side. Doors so large as to be discernible from afar; doors so small that few could find them; but even through the smallest there was the same ability to enter the treasure-hall. Travelers in those days might fear imagined ogres, jinn, and terrifying guardians to counter talismans; but the keys of safety were everywhere in hand, for all these beings were amenable to caresses the caresses of a heart which approached them with reverence and affection, asking questions but never injuring; always treating everything within the treasury (for it is living) as gently as one should approach to watch a sleeping babe.

It is for us ourselves not to pass these things by. If we did nothing more than study the *materia medica* of those days to see what products were available, we should have ample material for thought, and become cognizant of the links between that age and this. The drugs are still cultivated, and still used in the East in the manner of the past, and the history of their names adds to our understanding of their uses. While it is true we can supply our needs through an order to the apothecary based on information imparted to us through various intermediaries, we may some day find that in doing so we have omitted to look inside the treasure-house. To go back to the old paths, watching nature and studying the uses of the living plants, is not to lose the definite therapeutic effects we seek. Far from it; and there is the added insight into that universal life which needs transference from the inexhaustible abundance of nature at large into the thirsting lack of the patient in particular. It would then be not simply as a "relaxation" from the exacting labors of the city that one would go abroad into the country-side. It would be for the purpose of retiring to watch, and meditate upon the manifestations of the quiet persistent surging life of creatures below the level of man, thereby to learn something of the secret through which the equilibrium of health is to be restored to the needy and also oneself—to receive from the fountains of life.

Dietetic Treatment

In these days, this form of treatment is increasingly to the fore. But whereas modern thought is in terms of food-values and the like, *The Canon* insists (and rightly) on the necessity for studying physiological and psychological incompatibilities in regard to each component of the diet, and for selecting the various articles of food according to their constitution, so that they shall be in harmony with the constitution of the patient.

Regiminal Treatment

The term "regimen" has a wide range. This has already been sufficiently indicated at the end of Part Three.[32] The consideration of the specific constitution of the patient, of his present state, and of the conditions which are likely to arise during the various successive phases of his illness, must pervade every detail of the prescription of the regimen, to ensure that the correspondences between the state and the various measures adopted shall throughout be as harmonious as possible.

In this way, the great importance of individual artistry in treatment is constantly insisted on, by contrast with the prevalent stereotyping of therapeutic methods, whether in regard to state regulated practice in its various branches, or in the provision of medical relief on a wholesale scale, or in the efforts to subject as much as possible to the output of team-work. The atmosphere thus created helps the student to realize that the last word has not been said when the clinician's discourse over the hospital bed is ended, and the protocols, and therapeutic orders have been set upon the bed sheet.

The following may be quoted here, from Bauer:[33]

> "It is true, there is a difference between the pure medical science and the art of its practical application at the patient's bedside. This art is somewhat more, indeed, than this application; it requires more than a complete knowledge of all scientific details; it is and will be always an art which never will be transformed into an exact science, as the complete understanding of one person's psychophysical machinery never will permit us to understand a second man's personality just as well by a pure analogy, because of the practically infinite variability of the individual constitution. The individual analysis must start always anew, and what science of the human constitution may help, is only to establish certain groups of more or less pronounced common characteristics . . . it will never replace entirely the doctor's art to . . . take the individual particularities of his patient into consideration . . . in constructing his diagnosis and in applying the fitted treatment."

The clinical handling of a case is guided from time to time by the experience which has been concentrated into aphorisms. Like many; ancient medical works, The Canon abounds in these also, and some of them will not doubt be found among the modern collections of aphorisms which are available. In this way, too, it may be true to say that the conduct of a modern case sometimes receives the personal guidance of the wisdom of the past.

Progress

Progress[34] is a relative term. The common error is to assume that it is an end in itself. Things which can be described as "up to date," or cast aside as "out of date," do not belong to the real basis of human life. The idea of progress is associated with the introduction of mechanical improvements of all kinds; with mass production of manufactured articles; with the standardization of existence. In the domain of medicine, it is more particularly associated with an increasing knowledge of concrete facts, with specific discoveries in etiology and treatment; and with a new nomenclature.

To illustrate the relative character of "progress" one may call to mind that many discoveries and inventions are simply actualizations of ideas previously current among thinkers, but perhaps not noticed at the time, or even repudiated or attacked as heretical. Further, as to the changes in nomenclature which occur as time goes on: because our language and idiom is different, many are apt to think the old statements were necessarily incorrect. In medieval books dealing with *materia medica*, they said for instance: "dissolved in vinegar, the action is so-and-so," whereas we say simply: acetum, action and uses: . . . In chemistry, they might say "fire produces YZ," whereas we says "on heating Z, the result is Y and X." In medical text-books there are innumerable diseases which are not mentioned in old works; and some diseases of the old books do not appear in modern ones. This is partly explained by the undoubted fact that we have diseases which once did not exist, whereas other conditions, very common in those days, certainly never occur now. The methods of teaching are different. In these days we convey information much more quickly and readily by diagrams, charts, tables, styles of print, not to mention experiments,.and moving-pictures. This fact does not prove that the learning of those days, acquired so laboriously, was faulty.

That which is called "progress" is also sometimes merely "fashion." The search for an elixir of life, for instance, has not ceased in the least. The gland therapy for restoring youth is perhaps the most conspicuous of modern variants of ancient research. Cupping and venesection were habitually used solely with the idea of "keeping fit" they have given place to the vogue of athletics and sport. New treatments for various conditions are introduced from time to time, and seem to be great advances because they are often conspicuously successful at first. How often do they not give place to still newer methods, and perhaps finally pass into entire oblivion? The fashion changes, and the old, is supplanted.

It will be suggested that knowledge is not simply "acquaintance with an assemblage of facts" and that facts in the aggregate do not suffice to constitute "truth."[35] There is a tendency to extol the acquisition of facts, as "adding to the sum of knowledge," and as being evidence of "progress." There are different forms of knowledge: human, angelic, divine. The perfection of knowledge is wisdom. There are different forms of truth: scientific, logical, moral, ontological, philosophical, theological, etc. But as to "Ultimate Truth," this is humanly unattainable, as may be illustrated by the accompanying diagram.

The observer and the thing observed are shown in plan, as being separated by a straight semi-transparent screen. The letters A to I represent the position of as many observers. For the purpose of illustration these are supposed to be of different nationalities and not necessarily acquainted with one another's language; they also belong to different periods of life (childhood, youth, etc.). The observer at A may be supposed only to be able to see the part of the object marked A; the observer at B. similarly, may only be able to see the part marked B. and so on. But even if any of the observers could see several parts, evidently there still remain some areas which are out of the range of vision of all persons, as marked K. L, M. No one can comprehend the whole, under the restrictions given.[36]

This conception may be applied to the interpretation of terms applied even to familiar objects. In studying The Canon, for instance, it is not enough to know the dictionary equivalent of an Arabic or Latin word, for the full meaning is not always adequately conveyed thereby. The word "*akhlat*" may be taken as an example. It is rendered humour, humour, body-fluid, juice. The impression conveyed by each equivalent varies according to ideas commonly associated with the word and the circumstances under which we first heard it. The conception of the word humour was necessarily different in the mind of the ancient Greek physician, of the Hindu sage. of the erudite Chinese, of the alchemist of the Middle Ages, of the characters in Shakespeare, of the modern laity, of the student of esotericism, and of the modern bio-chemist.

It has been said that we shall reach Truth by whatever road we take. But this is not so. There is really only one path which will take us there direct. All the others are devious and arduous, and in t he end only bring us to the confines of Truth. We may trace out every separate road as outlined for us by as many separate thinkers of the past or present; we may pursue the highway which modern science has opened out; we may decide also to study the tracks with which we are furnished by nature itself. But even after all these have been slowly and laboriously surveyed by spiritual insight, the best we can attain is but the fringe of Reality.

The Relation Between *The Canon* and Modern Thought

Considerations[37] are not wanting which entitle The Canon of Medicine of Avicenna to an esteemed position in modern thought. In the first place, there is the outstanding intellectual culture of the [Islamic] Empire—during the period of history to which Avicenna belongs. Secondly, in the case of much of his teaching, it may be said that the difference from ours is largely only that his speech is alien and is apt to be misunderstood. In these days, the great complexity of the language with which we express our scientific thought corresponds with the intricacy of the instruments wherewith facts are elicited. Thirdly, many of the advances of modern times offer the solutions to the very theorems and propositions of former times. Finally, ideas are to be found in his work which provide suggestions for useful research in the future.

The importance of idea over material achievement is not to be forgotten. The achievements of any age are subject to decay with the lapse of centuries but the ideas which gave rise to them remain living through all cycles. Therefore to propose a real place for Avicenna in modern thought is not to propose a return as it were to old architecture, or the costumes of long ago. It is rather to render accessible today the picture which he painted and so enable it to renew its still vital message. It is to play over again the music which he expressed and enable perhaps one or two to rejoice in it. And this without obscuring the issue by discussing nationality or schools of thought or evolution of ideas or technical methods.

If it appear to some a fault that the master appears to have used passages from other works and this without full acknowledgment, it should be remembered that after all a painter may use pigments which someone else has manufactured and is allowed even to employ other persons (usually pupils) to execute certain portions of his picture. Indeed, even after his decease, it is not improper that some may have been entrusted with the delicate task of touching up faded portions of the canvas which he bequeathed.

The place for Avicenna in modern thought is gained when it is agreed that he shall be viewed as one who entered this world entrusted with a mission independently to express for that age, by means of those various tools which he then found in it, the wisdom which is unchanging and impersonal. So also there is the need today that this same wisdom should be re-expressed for this age by means of the new data which lie to our hands.

The Intellectual Culture Contemporary with Avicenna

Carra de Vaux, in his monograph Avicenna[38] furnishes particularly striking comments, as follows:

"The more we investigate the enormous literary output of the [Islamic] empire and come into intimate appreciation of the master minds of the middle epoch and of antiquity, the more we become aware of their sincerity.

"We should, we think, offer our salutations to these great personalities of that day whose works and lives were equally encyclopedic.

"Our own times do not show more worthy figures; we complacently assume that there are no more worthy than ourselves because science, so greatly developed today, cannot be held all within one single head. That may be. But it is only right to admit that science has less unity and harmony today than formerly it had; that it is less pure than it was under the grand peripatetic discipline. Our attitude towards that is neither humble nor sincere.

"In these days we are concerned too much to have our name blazoned forth than to grasp a great extent of science. We are more anxious to uphold the profession than to have a passion for study; we seek titles and reputation rather than real know-ledge; and in order to appear more specialized than our ancestors wet expose ourselves to the judgment of posterity as having smaller minds and fettered souls."

As to the state of civilization in the western Saracen empire we have the very illuminating description of Ameer Ali,[39] "The Muslims covered the countries where they settled with networks of canals. To Spain they gave the system of irrigation by flood-gates, wheels and pumps. Whole tracts of land which now lie waste and barren were covered with olive groves, and the environs of Seville alone, under Muslim rule, contained several thousand oil factories. They introduced the staple products, rice, sugar, cotton, and nearly all the fine garden and orchard fruits, together with many less important plants, like ginger, saffron, myrrh, etc. They opened up the mines of copper, sulphur, mercury, and iron. They established the culture of silk, the manufacture of paper and other textile fabrics; of porcelain, earthenware, iron, steel, leather. The tapestries of Cordova, the woolen stuffs of Myrcia, the silks of Granada, Almeria, and Seville, the steal and gold work of Toledo, the paper of Salibah, were sought all over the world. The ports of Malaga, Carthage, Barcelona and Cadiz were vast commercial emporia for export and import. In the days of their prosperity, the Spanish Muslims maintained a merchant navy of more than a thousand ships. They had factories and representatives on the Danube. With Constantinople they maintained a great trade which ramified from the Black Sea, and the eastern shores of the Mediterranean into the interior of Asia, and reached the ports of India and China, and extended along the African coast as far as Madagascar.

> "In the midst of the tenth century, when Europe was about in the same condition that Caffraria is now, enlightened Moors, like Abul Cassem were writing treatises on the principles of trade and commerce. In order to supply an incentive to commercial enterprise, and to further the impulse to travel, geographical registers, gazetteers, and itineraries were published under the authority of the government, containing minute descriptions of the places to which they related, with particulars of the routes and other necessary matters. Travelers like Ibn Battuta visited foreign lands in quest of information, and wrote voluminous works on the people of those countries, on their fauna and flora, their mineral products, their climate and physical features, with astonishing perspicacity and keenness of observation.
>
> "The love of learning and arts was by no means confined to one sex. The culture and education of the women proceeded on parallel lines with that of the men and women were as keen in the pursuit of literature and as devoted to science as men. They had their own colleges;[40] they studied medicine and jurisprudence, lectured on rhetoric, ethics, and belles-lettres and participated with the stronger sex in the glories of a splendid civilization. The wives and daughters of magnates and sovereigns spent their substance in founding colleges and endowing universities, in establishing hospitals for the sick, refuges for the homeless, the orphan and the widow."

Cordova was the most celebrated western university of the Empire at the time of Avicenna. This is well known as an instance of the high degree of culture of the day. Ameer Ali speaks of "that wonderful kingdom of Cordova, which was the marvel of the Middle Ages, and which when all Europe was plunged in barbaric ignorance and strife alone held the torch of learning and civilization bright and shining before the western world."[41] The greatness of the city is indicated by its population which is given by Haeser[42] as 300,000, and by Campbell[43] as one million; and by the library of "about 200,000" volumes.

To see the city today, traversed as it can be from wall to wall, within half an hour on foot, and to read of an extent of "twenty-four miles one way and six in the other"[44] shows that the word "kingdom" conveys a truer idea of its greatness. To read of "innumerable libraries, 3,800 mosques, 60,000 palaces and mansions, 200,000 houses inhabited by the common people, 3700 baths, 80,000 shops, besides hostels and caravanserais" is to wonder how so much can have come to be now represented by so little ("every dwelling-place, even if it has been blessed ever so long, will one day become a prey."[45] Nevertheless, the "grand mosque" alone, which is still at any rate externally intact (and interiorly is still surely one of the wonders of the world despite its mutilation) stands sponsor for the rest; and no doubt many of the existing imposing buildings—now devoted to very different uses—stand for the palaces and mansions. As to the literary treasures, these have been traced at least in part from Spain to Fez, as shown by Horne,[46] with the Roud El Qartas as his authority; and he then points to years of pilfering from the library of the great mosque of El Karouiyan at Fez, as having scattered these works forever.

A study of the street names, and even the place names and current dialect in "Moorish Spain" today also confirms the story of past greatness. But the mystical knowledge displayed in the dispositions of the decorative designs and their poetic inscriptions on the walls of the Alhambra halls, state-rooms, and private apartments can leave no doubt of unsurpassed artistic power where every sense impression was deliberately drawn on. Lights and shadows and colors changing with the-hours of the day; musical effects of simultaneous diversity of disposition of flowing water; perfumes; courting of the prevailing breezes; interior architectural form; and furnishings, animate and manufactured—all these were combined for the achievement of a perfect representation of (divine, over and above human) beauty.

Among the Chinese? The bearing of Chinese philosophical thought on the subject of Avicenna lies in the fact that we here meet with a notable example of intimacy of relation between world conception and medicine. The writings which are so carefully studied today by so many sinologists were extant at the time of Avicenna, and are still held in the highest esteem by Chinese thinkers. The modern Chinese philosopher is supposed to say to the westerner, "What is the reason for which you deem yourselves our betters? Have you excelled us in arts or letters?

Have our thinkers been less profound than yours? Has our civilization been less elaborate, less complicated, less refined than yours? Why, when you lived in caves and clothed yourselves with skins, we were a cultured people . . . ."[47]

The attitude towards western learning so displayed may be blamed by many, but is certainly praised by those who have studied the philosophy most deeply. As long ago as 1876 we read conclusive evidence.[48] If some students discuss their philosophy with a certain cynicism,[49] others[50] see into the justice of their conceptions. As Caruso remarks: "We need not be blind to the many errors and absurdities of the ancient occultism to understand and grant the truth that underlies its system."[51] These words are exactly applicable to *The Canon of Medicine* of Avicenna.

It should be added that errors and absurdities are apt to be ascribed to ancient authors which really arose from misunderstandings and ignorance on the part even of contemporary pupils. The subsequent generations perpetuated the errors, and even in these days the attempt to represent the real meaning of ancient texts by translations exposes one to unexpected extraordinary pitfalls. Our idiom is so diverse from the technical Chinese.

The Nature of the Knowledge Presented by *The Canon*

The Canon is a precis and not a sum-total of Avicenna's knowledge. Numerous passages occur in *The Canon* which show that this is the case, that it is a series of notes or skeleton outlines of thought not too lengthy to be memorized by his students[52] much as they would memorize the Quran. Thus, "to the full extent necessary, and yet with apt brevity,"[53] "do not place in medicine what does not belong to it,"[54] "having discussed the equable temperaments sufficiently,"[55] "I purposely omit reference to certain other problems relative to the fluids of the body just as much as is necessary to enable you to practice medicine intelligently."[56] Many passages also refer to others of his own works for further details, to avoid confusing the purely medical issue of *The Canon*. These philosophical works are gradually becoming more widely known.

"Generally speaking, the saying of the saints and sages are terse, presenting only the germs of truth; these are developed by later teachers and then expanded and added to. We must see to it, however, that we get at the original meaning of the saints and sages."[57]

"Books are only words and the valuable part of words is the thought therein contained. That thought has a certain bias, which cannot be conveyed in words, yet the world values words as being the; essence of books. But though the world values them, they are not of value; as that sense in which the world values them is not the sense in which they are valuable."[58]

To say that a work is the product of the age in which an author lives is certainly often an error, for it is to confuse the person's insight with the tools (the language at his command) available to express himself with. Similarly to work out the relation between a literary work and the religious belief of the author, as for instance to show the relation between Islamic science and the Quran carries the same fallacy with it. The Prophet said, "Every soul when born is a faithful follower; it is afterwards that he becomes unfaithful"—which is to say that the form of religious belief is a secondary implantation, whereas the spirit of a sincere life can be traced to the original being.

Avicenna's medicine, like Indian medicine, has been traced to the Greek system. But it has been proved that the great works of *Charaka* and *Susruta* were available in Arabic, under the title of *Kitab shawshura al-Hindi*, from the 7th century.[59] Similarly, the view that the Chinese borrowed their philosophy of the five elements from the Turks has been sufficiently disposed of by Forke.[60] It is beside the purpose of this treatise to take up such questions.

The common notion that progress or stagnation in secular knowledge has a causal relationship with a certain religion is typically voiced in his address on "*Medicine and the Church*" by Sir Farquhar Buzzard.[61] The comment to make is: "*post hoc sed non propter hoc*." The advances in the science of medicine, as in all other sciences, are surely a part of the divine plan for mankind whereas the collateral abandonment of religious fundamentals remains a human responsibility.

The word "canon" (*qanun*): equivalent words: code of laws; series of principles; tao.[62] Principle is defined as "something antecedent, which exercises a real positive influence upon the consequent" = causes (four kinds, Avicenna) = reasons.

In view of this it is clear that *The Canon* is not properly to be regarded as an "encyclopedia" of the knowledge of the time, or to be contrasted, for instance, with the now classical "*Osler*."

The word "knowledge": knowledge is not simply an assemblage of "facts" nor is it to be made synonymous with "truth"—certainly not Absolute Truth, of which all human knowledge falls short although one single word is capable of containing or implying all knowledge, as in mathematics a single term may be equated with an infinite number of terms summed together. But even the mathematical sciences can only afford approximate truth.[63] We may recall the words, "If he attain to all knowledge, he is far off still."[64]

Facts, as St. Thomas[65] explains, are what our intellect regards as external objects—and as we judge of them only in terms of our sense organs—these objects may be different. God knows them as they are. Our intellect depends on our imagination and that depends on our senses. Our senses only convey discrete fragments which we gather into one continuous impression regardless of intervening points." We live as it were in a network only the nodes of which are evident to the senses.

Mystical Insight

There is a distinction between knowledge gained in the ordinary manner and that gained by "mystical insight" (*kashf*). The writer of *Gulshan-i-raz's*[66] advises his readers to follow this, saying:

> Straightway lift yourself above time and space,
> Quit the world and be yourself a world for yourself.
> And
>
> The moment we are enlightened within
> We go beyond the voidness of a world confronting us.
> —Seng-ts'an, quoted by Susuki.[67]

As this "opens up all of a sudden a world hitherto undreamed of, it is an abrupt and discrete leaping from one plane of thought to another."[68]

> Real science is seeing the fire directly,
> Not mere talk, inferring the fire from the smoke.
> Your scientific proofs are more offensive to the wise
> Than the urine and breath whence a physician infers.[69]

"Man looks at the surface of the ocean. Yet he is so small that he cannot even be compared to one of its drops, limited as he is in intellect and in his knowledge. It is only to those who, having just touched creation, bow to God, forgetting their limited self, that God has remained. These through whom God has spoken are the only beings who have been able to give any truth to the world."[70]

"The mind is not like a horizontal door which haste be made larger by force. You must clear away the obstructions arising from creaturely desire and then it will be pure and clear with no limit to its knowledge.

Heng Ch'u said, 'When the mind is enlarged it can enter into everything throughout the universe.' He who praises God knows about Him."[71]

This attitude towards nature is to be claimed for Avicenna on the plain evidence of his other writings including the *al-Najat* which appropriately appears in the Arabic version of *The Canon* printed at Rome in 1593 and of the Libellus on the powers of the hearts and is included in the Latin edition of *The Canon*, 1595.[72]

The acquisition of knowledge by this process demands nothing more than a keen observation of the life around us and was as much within his reach as ours. Such knowledge is not too restricted to one period of history, one language, or to one or two universities. And if it should seem that because our civilization is so different his opportunities were much less, we may pause to reflect that the difference between our age and his is chiefly one of mechanical appurtenances and phraseology; and that even to this day we need not travel far (i.e., the old streets of Cordova and Granada or more definitely, to northern Africa) to see much the same sort of scenery as he was accustomed to, much the same sort of life as is drawn in the 1001 Nights. In any case, what is human life, at bottom, but a matter of buying and selling, receiving and giving, seizing and relinquishing, constructing and demolishing, acquiring learning and losing it, seeking power and breaking it, bidding and forbidding, giving in marriage and seeking to obtain in marriage, birth and death.

The significant phrase "seeing into one's own nature,"[73] in which most admirable work occur many passages by way of explanation) gives a graphic description of that which gives Avicenna his superiority. *The Canon* is simply the medical garb in which the one Truth is expounded. It is for us also to perceive it in whatever idiom it might be described—western, eastern, Islamic, Confucian or Buddhist, for example.

It would then seem as if the mind were now able to float as it were round all the concepts the human being has ever given to the world, or round all the most familiar events of one's daily life, and perceive clearly that which can never be set forth in words. We should then also quote the words."[74] I perceive of it that it is something, but what it is I cannot perceive. Only it seems if I could conceive it, I should comprehend all truths.

Further than this, to find that some of the statements in *The Canon* are certainly erroneous and that modern investigations have placed us at an infinitely greater advantage, does not invalidate the work as a whole. Its possibilities for suggesting thoughts of real value today are more realized the more one reads between the lines, and the present treatise does not claim to exhaust them.

"Let not the authority of the writer offend thee, whether he be of title or great learning, but let the love or pure truth entice thee to read."[75]

Insight into eternal truths. A person may: (1) glimpse them; (2) understand them moderately; (3) understand them fairly thoroughly. But in describing them to another, he may explain them: (i) imperfectly (no one can explain them properly!); (ii) inadequately or incompletely; (iii) wrongly because of: (a) imperfect education; (b) educational bias; (c) religious or anti-religious bias; (d) inherently erroneous methods of thought; (e) restriction to logic. Such truths, again, may be denied by persons being told of them, for because in their turn they misunderstand, or understand only in part, either through careless attention, and (a) to (e).

Insight Versus Intuitional Knowledge

A note should here be made that the term "insight" as used here bears a rather different meaning to that pertaining to the term "intuitive knowledge," which St. Thomas[76] ascribes solely to the angelic mind, and defines as "the attainment of the truth of a thing at a single glance without the aid of reasoning."[77] On the other hand this mode of perceiving truths need not be disallowed a rudimentary commencement among the powers of the human soul, just as the "brute" mind must be allowed to contain rudiments of those high mental capacities which characterize the human being. Throughout all orders of creation, the lower are endowed with the scaffolding for the manifestation of successively more exalted capacities of the higher.

The Basic Difference between The Canon and Modern Medicine

The Canon treats of:

I. Speculative Medicine
   - Certain fundamental principles (cosmology, psychology, metaphysics)

II. Practical Medicine
   - A. Application of Speculative Medicine to the study of (i) health; (ii) disease (tendency, predisposition, threshold stage, declared disease; (iii) cessation of life.
   - B. Actual treatment of "disease" by: (i) regimen, (ii) drugs, (iii) operative interference.

Modern Medicine consists of:

A. Principles of Medicine: The application of the facts of chemistry, physics, anatomy, biology to the systematic description of innumerable "diseases" classified as far as possible on the basis of the microbic theory; symptomatology; etiology; diagnosis.

B. Practice of Medicine

 i) Laboratory work
 ii) Therapeutics, Pharmacology and Dietetics
 iii) Surgery
 iv) Gynecology and Obstetrics
 v) States of Medicine: Hygiene in all its ranches
 vi) Psychological Medicine: Treatment of insanity
 vii) Legal medicine, etc.

Modern medicine is based on the conception of the universe as a conglomeration of dead matter out of which, by some unexplainable process, life may become evolved in forms. To Avicenna the whole of the universe is the manifestation of a universal principle of life, acting through the instrumentality of forms. Or, again, in modern medicine, the forms are the source of life; to Avicenna they are the product of life. Space itself is an aspect of the one life.[78]

In this way the difference between Avicenna's conception of "principles," and that of modern medicine is easily shown. To the school boy "science" would consist of (a) bookwork and (b) laboratory work which his teachers would insist is the basis of (a). Similarly, the medical curriculum begins with lectures, although these are more and more inclined to become laboratory demonstrations; and goes on to laboratory and hospital work.

In short, Avicenna's medicine, and all ancient and traditional medicine, is intimately bound up with philosophy, to wit, that of human nature—a philosophy which proves to be virtually identical with "modern scholastic philosophy," no doubt partly because the Quranic account of the origin of the human being tallies with the Christian.

Modern medicine, on the other hand, assuming the title and rank of a positive science, emphatically discards and excludes it. Hence we read: "the physiologist" (said Burdon Sanderson) "can pursue philosophy if he has a turn for it, but must understand that the moment he enters the field of philosophy he leaves his tools behind him." For "it is unfortunate that the limitations of scientific thought were often ignored by men of science in their writings . . . the result diverts those who know, but befogs the unsuspicious reader who will probably put the blame on his intelligence."[79]

"According to positivism, science cannot be as Aristotle conceived it, the knowledge of things through their ultimate causes, since material and formal causes are unknowable, final causes are illusions, and efficient causes are simply invariable antecedents, while metaphysics under any form is illegitimate."[80] Or, expressed more boldly, "philosophy" is considered to be the exact antithesis of the truth which modern medicine gives us, and is therefore inherently inadmissible to medicine.

The ignorance which accounts for this attitude is only met by insisting on proper definitions of terms. The following apply here:

Philosophy is "the science which is concerned with first causes and principles; it is the profound knowledge of the universal order, and the duties which that order imposes on the human being.[81]

Again, philosophy is the true perception and understanding of cause and effect. Metaphysics is "that portion of philosophy which treats of the most general and fundamental principles underlying all reality and all knowledge."[82] Psychology is "the science which treats of the soul and its operations" and, therefore, clearly, must be the real foundation of medicine.

It is in modern scholastic philosophy that the student finds ample exposure of the fallacy in positivism and its cognates, enabling him to detect the difference between false and true, expressed with enough force of logic to satisfy the most meticulous. This queen of all the sciences amply proves positivist science (including medicine) to be incomplete knowledge when taken alone. The knowledge of movement or change must be supplemented by mathematical and metaphysical viewpoints.[83] Such men as Albertus Magnus and Roger Bacon were convinced of the necessity of linking the sciences with philosophy.[84]

When medicine has in this way become ennobled it reaches its highest degree of perfection, in that it penetrates to the very depths of reality,85 admitting this knowledge to need, even then, a further complement to make it complete-namely, knowledge in relation to God ("Christian wisdom").

> *"Sapientia est scientia qua considerat causas primas et universales causas. Sapientia causas primas omnium causarum considerat."86 "Ille qui cognoscit causam altissimam simpliciter, qua est Deus dicitur sapiens simpliciter, in quantum per regulas divinas omnia potest judicare et ordinare."[87] "Non acquiritur studio humano, sed est deursum scendens."[88] "Cum homo per res creatas Deum cognoscit, magis videtur hoc perti nere ad scientiam, ad quam perti net formaliter, qu am ad*

sapientiam ad qu am pertinet materialiter: et e converso cum secundum res divinas judicamus de rebus creatis, magis hoc ad sapientiam quam ad scientiam pertinet."[89]

As St. Thomas said in his day, "they think that nothing exists besides visible creatures." [N.B.:"Creatures" are (a) animate; and (b) inanimate]. "They think that things proceed not by the divine will but by natural necessity."[90] So even in those days time and fortune were expended on researches which sound philosophy would have shown to be inherently futile.

We may reflect for instance on the reiterated search for a location of the soul, which the pioneer anatomists prosecuted, and also on the commonly repeated announcement to successive students of anatomy that the pineal gland is now no longer regarded as the site of the soul. There is the sub-conscious suggestion to the student that scientific research has effectively disposed of the medieval belief in the soul, whereas history only proves that the revolt against the precise teachings of the Council of Trent necessarily came to naught.[91] The very definition of "soul" which this council laid down makes a search for its location ludicrous.

Conceptions Known to Modern Medicine; but Not to Avicenna

Among the most important of these are: (1) the anatomy of the circulation of the blood. (2) the rate of that circulation. (3) The details found in The Canon's anatomy; the microscopic anatomy; such complexities as form the theme of Bayliss' Physiology. These details might be expressed as those of "the mechanics of the body." (4) Interactions in the tissues: chemical and cellular metabolism. (5) In pathology: the microbic theory; the endless and always increasing number of "diseases"; the laboratory diagnosis of dysfunction of organs; (albuminuria was, of course, unknown); symptoms as evidences of disordered reflexes. (6) In treatment: the use of antisera and specific anti-substances of organisms; hypodermic medication; complex drug treatment has passed out of vogue; surgery.

Considerations which suggest that these instances of ignorance are not as grave as is supposed, and do not invalidate the standing of ancient medicine in regard to actual practice.

Circulation of a kind was propounded in the case of the "breath," the elements, and the body-fluids, though not along anatomical channels. The Chinese recognized a process of "revolution," a succession of cyclical changes an ebb and flow. Indeed, it is suggested in *Duhalde*[111] that the Chinese knew of the circulation of the blood itself some hundred years BC.

Wieger,[112] discussing whether the Chinese knew of the circulation of the blood twenty centuries before Harvey or not, decides truly that "their knowledge of the circulation of the blood in the human microcosm was intuitive, not experimental, conjectured in imitation of the circulation of the vital principle in the universal microcosm, in which they believed. They guessed the fact, and they never verified it. . . . During more than twenty centuries, the how of the guessed circulation never worried their mind. The yin-yang circulates in a ring, the five agents do the same, the blood the same. That is all . . ." But if a doctrine which is common to Taoism and esotericism [that of microcosm and macrocosm] is allowed to be valid, the words "intuitive knowledge" cannot be made synonymous with "conjecture," "guess."

The rapidity of the changes was certainly not realized. The Chinese apparently believed that the circulation was completed only fifty times in one day. There is however room for fallacious.

Lest there should be over-satisfaction with ourselves, it may be suggested that the rapidity of the movement of the lymph was not realized before about 1908, and is perhaps not fully realized by many practitioners today; the rapidity of passage of food-materials down the small intestine was not known until the advent of the "bismuth" meal. The circulation of nerve-impulses is not yet admitted.

The capillaries of the liver are referred to[113] in the body in general.[114] True, what Avicenna calls capillaries are larger than those we see with the microscope. But he knew that the blood passes from large trunks into the liver, traverses "capillaries" in the liver, and re-emerges by large trunks.

Interactions in the tissues were conceived of as taking place with an ebb and a flow (which is correct); lymph exudes into the tissue-spaces. Interactions take a considerable time (true). Digestion goes on within the blood-vessels in various parts of the body.

Fermentation was the counterpart of bacterial growth as we know it. The term is used sufficiently specifically in the text.[115] Diseases were regarded chiefly as parts of a process; and there were but few processes (which is quite true: nine processes).116 Urinalysis was carried out in order to assess the functional state of the liver.[117]

Modern medicine claims its title to superiority by its successes, and judges the medicine of the past by its failures. But what would the judgment be if this method were reversed? Suppose we accepted the verdict of those among the laity (who are not so few) who are dissatisfied with their experiences of orthodox medicine and have turned to the "unqualified" of one kind or another, or those of other countries who prefer their native doctors still, or even those Europeans who have experienced triumphant success from native doctors, aver modern methods had failed? After all the ancient medicine is still practiced from Cairo to Calcutta, and a medicine not very different holds sway through the Far East. The late Sir Charles Pardy Lukis[118] is quoted as saying "Many of the empirical methods of treatment adopted by *hakims* are of the greatest value, and there is no doubt whatever that their ancestors, ages ago, knew many things which are nowadays being brought forward as new discoveries.[119]

Drug-treatment

The complexity of prescriptions of former times has given place to simple and short ones, and the tendency is to discard them altogether. But the reasons for the ancient method are given in the Canon, and Avicenna's choice of remedies depended on a careful consideration of the constitution of the remedies, as well as of the patient and his idiosyncrasies. Thus, certain ingredients would be allowed or disallowed in a given standard confection according to the nature of the particular patient. " The presence or absence, and the amount, of *nardus*, ginger, fennel-seed, anise, piper, *cyperus rotundus*, must be according to the season, and the age of the patient.[120]

F. Hartmann[121] describes the accuracy of native diagnosis[122] as "disconcerting," and describes certain forms of treatment (auto-chemotherapy, Bier treatment) as being practiced in a manner only different in outward appearance from the technique which we pride ourselves as being absolutely the "latest." "No wonder," he says, "that the Chinese are proud of their art, considering how long they have known that which we have only recently discovered." (These words can be fully endorsed, if only from a study of the Chinese classic on the pulse, Wan K'an t'ang, 80 volumes, discussed under the heading "*The Pulse*" in the present treatise.[123] Among other ancient Chinese medical works-first seen by the present writer in the very extensive collection in the Library of McGill University-reference may be made to the astonishing accuracy of representations of medicinal and other plants, and the almost dramatic representations of various diseases states in the *I tsung chin ch'un* by Hung Chou, extant in Avicenna's time. This work was reprinted between 1904 and 1924 and an older edition is in the Library of the *School of Oriental Studies*).

The cynical mind cannot be upheld which passes off the reputed successes during the Middle Ages as coincidences, and overlooks the modern crowded out-patient departments as evidences of the limitations of our current therapy and theory; nor can the skeptic be much noticed who denies miraculous cures rather than admit scientific theories to be in any sense inadequate.

Nevertheless, it is obvious that the principles of *The Canon* could not be taught over a hospital bed or in the out-patient department. It is true that they cannot cater for the wholesale requirements of the hospital or clinic. It should be clear to the candid that our modern technique does not avail for 100 per cent of cases; for those who do not benefit at least an experiment with other systems of treatment should not be denied. If the fault is laid at the feet of over-strenuous routine work, the more leisured may yet find an advantage in a system which puts the details of a person's constitution in all its aspects into the forefront, where there is no question of teaching it either to classes or even to possibly indifferent individuals. The words of Paracelsus may be recalled, where he says: a the doctor who loves his art does not undertake twenty cases but five, knowing that no one person can conscientiously treat more than a certain number. No one person could ever make the whole world sound."

Knowledge Common to Avicenna and Modern Medicine

A perusal of the text of The Canon will show many passages which apply quite well, without explanation, in these days. Thus, the following may be specified: the close relation between emotions and physiological states (shown to be even closer than modern research has realized); the classification of people into sanguine, phlegmatic, bilious, saturnine, frigid, "hot"; the physiology of sleep; and how posture may remedy insomnia.

Choice of Location for Dwellings

Health resorts. Climactic influences on health and illness- Plethoric maladies. Dietetics. Hydrotherapy. Regiminal treatment. The uses of counter-irritation. Bier treatment. The introduction of remedies into the urethra. The use of vaginal tampons. The use of anesthetics by the mouth (medicated wines: scopolamine). Testing the strength of a drug by animal experiment. The treatment of insanity by malaria.[124]

No doubt the great difference between the ancient and modern is one of outlook, which accounts for the difference of topic. That which appeared interesting and even important in those days is passed over by modern physiology and pathology. Each century has its own interests.

The mistake made is to suppose that the older interests were "wrong," "incorrect," "useless"; and to label them as "out of date." True, fashions of all kinds come to be out of date, but the epithets "right," "wrong" do not apply. The more carefully we observe modern science the more evident does it become that just its terminology and subject of conversation is different Things are seen from new angles, and things only surmised at then are amenable to tangible description now.

In fact, there occur moments, even at this day, when suggestive thoughts might be drawn from The Canon, to help in studying the individual, tedious, or baffling case, especially where the practice is far distant from the laboratories and appliances of modern medicine.

Of Interest to the Scholar

The present translation is based on the Latin versions published at Venice in 1608 and 1595, supported by a study of the Arabic edition printed at Rome in 1593 and the Bulaq edition.

It is true that as E. G. Browne pointed out, "The Latin Qanun swarms with barbarous words which are not merely transcriptions, but in many cases almost unrecognizable mistranscriptions of Arabic originals,"[125] and that Hirschberg and Lippert[126] regard the Latin as almost unintelligible, though they admit the "slavish adherence" of the Latin to the Arabic. Campbell[127] states that there was a "society of translators" at Toledo, about 1130 A.D., "whose method of translating from Arabic to Latin was to put the Latin equivalent over the Arabic words, disregarding the sense of the original." It is true that in many passages the obscurity is similar to the effect which would result if one were at this day to render idiomatic French word for word into English.

It is important to point out that the Latin of Volume I is very different from that of Vols. III-V; so different that the translation must have been the work of different persons. While the criticisms are justified with regard to these three volumes, they do not apply to the first, whose Latin is very close to the Arabic, and hardly to be improved. The difficulty really is that the Arabic itself is so condensed that the meaning can only be clearly represented in English by the use of many more words, whether to help out the meaning itself, or to make a presentable reading.

It may well be said, as did E. G. Browne, "He who judges Arabian Medicine only by the Latin translation will inevitably undervalue it and do it a great injustice. Indeed it is difficult to resist the conclusion that many passages in the Latin version of the *Qanun* of Avicenna were misunderstood or not understood at all by the translator, and consequently can never have conveyed a clear idea to the reader."[128]

The following aids to clearness have been utilized: (1) the study of Avicenna's other works, and of contemporary philosophical writings, in the existing translations. (b) The study of various Latin terms as understood by modern scholastic philosophy in its exposition of the medieval nomenclature. (c) The use of modern terms when there is no reasonable doubt of their referring to the same idea, though the literal term in the Latin is obsolete. The careful study of the original Arabic has here been of special importance, for words in the Latin version, which are evidently technical there, become merely colloquial when translated into English, whereas in the Arabic version, such words at once take on their proper character in the Arabic-English and Persian-English dictionaries (d) The use of tabulation of the matter. There are instances where this proves possible without omitting even a single Arabic word. (e) The use of paraphrase for certain passages. These are marked (p). A certain freedom of rendering has been inevitable in view of the importance of bringing the meaning of the text to the reader's notice without subjecting him to the need of reflecting deeply on passage after passage-as is requisite with the original Arabic (to have dealt with the work from the point of literature would have entailed giving the preference to safeguarding against likely criticisms at the hands of pure scholarship).

The main purpose of this treatise will now be seen to center in the idea that in the ancient philosophy there is material capable of useful application to-day. The selection of the work of Avicenna is not intended to provide an apologium for that one author, but is specially appropriate for these reasons: (i) his acknowledged excellence; (ii) his greater accessibility among medieval medical writings; (iii) a certain indefinable charm of expression peculiar to himself; but above all, (iv) the fact that his central theme is a conception of the nature of the human being really identical with that of Thomistic philosophy, and in these days specially stressed and developed by "modern scholastic philosophy." As these are related, so might Avicenna be related to a modern scholastic medicine, which would aim at reasons for health and ill health far deeper than those given by the microbic and cognate theories.

With Mercier,[129] "We do not regard the Thomistic philosophy . . . as a boundary which sets limits to personal activity of thought . . . but make use of his" (in this case, Avicenna's) "teaching as a starting-point from which we may go further afield."

With Maher,[130] we ". . . resuscitate and" (apply to medicine) ". . . a psychology that has already survived four and twenty centuries, and has had more influence on human thought and human language than all other psychologies together. My desire, however, has been not merely to expound, but to expand this old system . . . to make clear to the student of modern thought that this ancient and traditional psychology (and medicine) is not so absurd, nor these old thinkers as foolish, as current caricatures of their teaching would lead one to imagine. . . . To trespass (on the soul) . . . . is assumed by (many writers) to be the gravest of professional delinquencies."

Therefore Avicenna is allowed once more to present his theme. To the questions we are constrained to ask of him, we find our answers: (1) in his other writings; (2) in contemporary literature; (3) in the writings of modern Eastern thinkers; (4) in the works of St. Thomas; (5) in modern scholastic philosophy. If some truths are crudely expressed or perhaps faultily explained, it is our privilege to re-express and re-explain with those aids.

Those who may have failed to identify one single Truth under different garbs are not obliged to accord these garbs an unfriendly reception upon the stage of our modern world. To recall a favorite Indian metaphor, the danseuse has so robed herself, and displays such diversities of art that under the ever-changing colored beams of light it is difficult to believe there can be only one and the same artiste before us. Should it prove impossible to verify this, at least the very exhibition of the art should serve so to refresh that we can resume our work and ambitions with an added zest now confident that the future realization of our desires is not so intangible as at first appeared.

I deemed life was tranquillity and rest,
I find it but a never-ending quest;
And I, who sat in quietude and peace,
Toil on a journey that shall never cease
(Shamshad)

Why should the Cosmos turn its wheel of worlds
If not to search for Thee eternally?
Why should the tireless Sun arise each morn
If not to look for Thee?
(Zauq)

How can I win that Hidden One
Who sits within the secret place,
For even in my very dreams
She wears the veil upon Her face.

(Jurat)

For long, throughout the world, I sought for Thee,
Through weary years and ages of unrest—
At last I found Thee hidden in my arms
Within my breasts.

(Zauq)

That which is spread before us, beneath the unceasing surge and change of the crowded life of the thoroughfares of great cities, as well as beneath the panorama of nature herself, was surely understood by those who insisted " there is no second Cause," and by Chu Hsi in saying "the innumerable laws (of nature) all proceed from one source."[131] In this the thought is not pietistically of a Creator, but of a living Reality met (passively or receptively) or encountered (actively or contestingly) by us all at all times. That Reality must be understood before we handle the problem of our patient with real efficacy.

In the intention of this work, then, there comes into consideration that greater art of medicine—not an ethical Hippocratic ideal, but something of the divine—an art as real to Avicenna, philosopher, poet, musician, the worker among the great and the small, aware of the dramatic in life, as it should be to us. So we step out of the world of the modern critic, the scholar, and the medical historian, indeed of modern medicine itself, into one in which we stand, as it were, hand in hand, with the great Master of the East—almost with his very eyes gazing upon and scrutinizing this ever open book of life of ours—divested of the false notions of "progress" and "time." His language is thus no longer alien—and, incidentally, he lives again!

Avicenna's Preface

In the first place we render thanks to God, for the very excellence of the order of His creation, and the abundance of His benefits. His mercies are upon all the prophets. Secondly, is at the request of one of my special friends [was it al-Juzjani? LB], one whom I feel most bound to consider, that I prepare this book on medicine, setting forth its general and particular laws to the full extent necessary, and yet with apt brevity.

Volume I: General Medicine

My plan is to deal with the general aspects of each of the two divisions of medicine—the speculative and the practical. Then I shall treat of the general principles applicable to the diagnosis of the properties of the simples, following this with a detailed account of them. I shall, then, take up the disorders which befall each individual member, beginning with an account of its anatomy, and that of its auxiliary. The anatomy of the several members and their auxiliaries is dealt with in the first book. Having completed the account of the anatomy, I shall show how the health of the member is to be maintained.

This subject being completed, I proceed to a general discourse about general diseases: their causes, the signs by which they are recognized, and the modes of treatment. After this, I pass on to the special diseases and will point out in as many cases as possible: (1) the general diagnosis of their characters, causes and signs; (2) the special diagnostic features; (3) the general rules of treatment; (4) the special methods of treatment by (a) simples; and (b) compounded medicines.

I include specially designed tables under the subject of simples to enable you to survey the facts rapidly as to the adjuvants for treating disease by simples.

I have deemed it best to consider compounded medicines, their adjuvants, and how to mix them separately in a formulary. This it is my intention to compose after the special subjects are dealt with. Disorders not confined to one member are described in this book; cosmetics are spoken of, and the knowledge set forth in previous books is assumed. God helping me to complete this volume, the formulary will be added to it. Every follower of my teachings, who wishes to use them profitably, should memorize most of this work, even though he not understand it all.

It is my intention to prepare further volumes if God should prolong my life still further, and if circumstances prove propitious. [Avicenna was to complete five volumes of which this is the translation of the first volume. LB.]

...

A brief summary of the contents of remaining volumes, II, III, IV, and V of *The Canon* are: [Volumes I, II and V have been translated into English. LB]

Volume II: Simple Drugs

This volume gives a detailed material medical pharmacology and therapeutics of drugs. It has two parts.

Part One. General Principles: These deal with the temperament or constitution of drugs, and how it is determined: (1) by experiment; and (2) by deduction. Conditions of the experiment such as, its being on the human body, drug to be free of extrinsic and intrinsic alterations, the trial to be allopatric and made on simple diseases, drug to be qualitatively and quantitatively corresponding to the severity of the disease, etc., have been described. Part one also gives an account of all the actions which drugs may possess and describes the method of collection and preservation of the various herbal and other products.

Part Two. List of Drugs: It gives 797 drugs in seriatim according to the Abjad system. The properties of each drug have been described under the following headings: general description of the drug, tests for its purity, qualities, general and special actions on each system of the body or on special diseases; specific actions; antidotal properties; alternative remedies and adjuvants.

Volume III: Diseases of Individual Members

In Volume III, the various diseases have been discussed systematically, with their etiology, symptoms, diagnosis, prognosis and treatment with simple drugs. Special mention may be made of the following sections:

Head: brain, (intemperaments, headache in all its aspects, organic diseases of the brain, epilepsy, paralysis, etc.) eye, ear, nose, mouth, throat, and teeth. Chest: lungs, heart, breasts. Alimentary tract: stomach, intestines, liver, gall bladder and spleen. Intestines and the anus, disorders of the rectum. Urinary tract: the kidneys, bladder and urine. The male reproductive system; the female reproductive system, conception, pregnancy, and diseases of women. Muscles: joints, and feet.

Volume IV: General Diseases

Part One. Fevers: general description of fevers; their periodicity; causes such as constipation, diarrhea, dietetic indiscretion; excessive activity; excessive wakefulness; fear or anger; pain, inflammation, putrefaction, humoural disturbances; etc. Diagnosis of fevers; epidemic fevers; small pox; phthisis. Prognosis. Management of symptoms such as thirst, rigors, diarrhea, vomiting, sleeplessness, pain, headache, etc. Treatment of fevers: general and specific. Subject of crisis.

Part Two. Boils and swellings. Leprosy. Minor surgery. Wounds and their general treatment. Injuries: fractures and dislocations. Ulcers. Glandular swellings.

Part Three. Poisoning with mineral, vegetable and animal products. Bites from animals and man.

Part Four. Beauty culture. Leanness and obesity. Hair, nails and skin. Treatment of offensive odors and discolorations including leucoderma. Pediculosis. Pitting from small pox, etc.

Volume V: The Formulary

This volume gives details of special prescriptions and antidotes; their form such as pills, powders, syrups, decoctions, confections, elixirs, etc, and their method of preparation. A thorough discourse about laxatives; purgative and non-purgative powders; medicinal powders, dosages; electuaris; potions and thickened juices; jams and preserves; pills; greens and cereals; lotions; and ointments and dressings. Prescriptions for different diseases. Weights and measures.

Avicenna's Introduction

Medicine comprises two parts, one theoretical, and one practical, though both are really speculative science. That which is specially named theory relates to the formation of opinions and the showing of the evidence upon which they are based, without reference to the mode of acting upon them. Thus this part deals with the temperaments, the humours, the drives, and with the forms, the symptoms, and the causes of disease. That which is specially named practical relates to the mode of acting upon this knowledge, and the prescription of a regimen.

For instance, it is that part of medicine which helps us understand how the health of the body is to be maintained in this or that state, and by what means we can heal the diseases with which the body is afflicted. Practical does not refer to the performance of surgical operations. It is the art which teaches us in what way to procure healing— the healing art.

The human being takes its origin from two things: (1) the male semen, which plays the part of factor; and (2) the female menstrual discharge, which provides the matter.

Each of these is fluid and moist, but there is more wateriness and earthly substance in the female blood and female sperm, whereas air and fire are predominant in the male sperm. It is essential that at the outset of the congelation of the two components there should be moisture, even though earth and fire are found in the product. The earth provides the firmness and rigidity; the fire provides the maturative power. These give the coagulum (*"He created man from a clot"* Quran, 96:2) a certain hardness or firmness. But this hardness is not as great in degree as that possessed by a stone or glass. For these are either not soluble at all or only soluble to a degree imperceptible to our senses, however long one exposes them to solvents. Were the hardness comparable to this, the product of conception would never suffer injury however long or however persistently a solvent were applied. But that is not so. The act is contrary.

Our bodies are exposed to injury from two directions—externally and internally. The source of internal injury is the dissipation of the moisture from which we are created, and this dissipation proceeds in an orderly manner. The second source is the putrefactive breakdown and metamorphosis of the humour into a form such that the fermentative phenomena of life are no longer able to proceed.

The second source of injury differs from the first in that dryness is here introduced by virtue of depravity of humour; and this dryness continues neutralizing the moisture of the body until the form ceases to have a capacity for life.

Finally, the putrefactive breakdown disperses the vitality, because it first destroys the moisture and then disperses it, and simply dry ash is left behind.

Therefore we see that these two sources of destruction [of the living product of conception] are different from those arising from other causes —such as, freezing cold, torrid heat, grave forms of loss of continuity, various maladies. But it is in regard to the first two named sources of destruction that we find the more important factors relative to the question of the preservation of health.

Each of them takes its origin from extrinsic and intrinsic agents. The extrinsic agents are for example, the atmosphere, which is a solvent and putrefacient. The intrinsic agents are, for example, the innate heat, which is the agent within us through which moisture is dispersed: the extraneous heat generated within us from the aliments, and through other agents which cause putrefactive changes in the [native] moistures.

All these agents mutually aid one another in rendering the body dry. And yet it is true that our perfection and soundness and the power to perform our various actions depend on a degree of dryness of the blood. But the degree of dryness becomes relatively greater and greater until we die. Therefore, this dryness is inevitable.

If we were at the outset essentially composed of moisture, heat would have to overcome it or else the heat would be choked by it. Therefore the heat continues to exert its own effect, that is, it produces more and more desiccation. But whatever degree of dryness there might be at the outset (of life), it reaches equilibrium, and remains so until the limit of equilibrium in regard to dryness is reached. The heat remaining constant, the dryness is now relatively greater than before for the matter is less, and hence holds more.

Therefore it is not difficult to understand that the dryness passes on beyond the stage of equilibrium, and goes on steadily increasing until the whole of the moisture of the body is consumed. Therefore (we may say) that the innate heat is the cause of its own extinction, for it is itself the reason for its own matter being consumed. We may compare it to the flame of a lamp; the light goes out when all the matter has been used up.

As the dryness increases, the innate heat diminishes. The loss continues unceasingly till death, and the moisture which is lost is not restored. The loss goes on more and more.

The dryness (of the body) is increased in two ways: by lessening of the power of receiving matter; by lessening of the native moisture resulting from dispersal of the (innate) heat. The heat becomes more feeble because dryness predominates in the substance of the members, and because the innate moisture becomes relatively less. The innate moisture is to the innate heat as the oil of a lamp is to the flame. For there are two forms of moisture in the flame: water, which holds its own, and oil, which is used up. So, in a corresponding manner, the innate heat holds its own in respect of the innate moisture, but is used up *pari passu* with increase of extraneous heat, due, for example, to defective digestion, which is comparable with the aqueous moisture of the flame. As the dryness increases, the innate heat lessens, and the result is natural death.

For the reason why the (human) body does not live any longer than it does lies in the fact that the initial innate moisture holds out against being dispersed both by the alien heat and by the heat in the body itself (both that which is innate and that derived from bodily movement). And this resistance is maintained as long as the one is weaker than the other, and as long as something is provided to replace that which has been thus dispersed, to wit, from the aliment. Furthermore, as we have already stated, the power or drive which operates upon the aliment in order to render it useful in this way only does so up to the end of life.

Therefore, we may say that the art of maintaining health is not the art of averting death or of averting extraneous injuries from the body or of securing the utmost longevity possible to the human being. It is concerned with two other things: (1) the prevention of putrefactive breakdown; and (2) the safeguarding of innate moisture from too rapid dissipation and maintaining it at such a degree of strength that the original type of constitution peculiar to the person shall not change even up to the last moment of life.

This is secured by a suitable regimen, namely: (a) one which will ensure the replacement of the innate heat and moisture which are dispersed from the body as exactly as possible; and (b) a regimen which will prevent any agents which would lead to a rapid dessication from gaining the upper hand excluding agents which produce a normal desiccation; (c) one which safeguards the body from the development of putrefactive processes within it and from the influence of alien heat (whether extraneous or intrinsic) because all bodies have not the same degree of innate moisture and innate heat. There is a great diversity in regard to them.

Moreover, every person has his own term of life, during which the desiccation inevitable to his temperament (constitution) and the degree of innate heat, and of innate moisture can be withstood.

Nevertheless, factors may arise which assist desiccation, or are injurious in some other way. For which reason, many assert that the former are natural causes of death, whereas the latter are accidental. And under this view, the art of maintaining health consists in guiding the body to its natural span of life by paying attention to whatever things conduce thereto. There are two drives to be fostered by the doctor in striving for this object: (1) the nutritive drive whereby that is replaced which is constantly being lost to the body namely earthiness and aquosity; and (2) the sensitive drive (animal faculty), that is, the pulsatile faculty which is concerned with the replacement of that which is lost to the body by the breath namely air and fire. And since aliments are only potentially like the thing nourished, an alternative drive had to be created so that they could be changed actually into the likeness of the thing nourished. In this way the aliment becomes effective.

The instruments and channels necessary for this had to be created also—namely the means by which material is attracted, expelled, retained, and digested (sequence by sequence, turn by turn).

Therefore, we may say that the essential considerations in the art of preserving the health consist in maintaining equilibrium between all these various concomitant factors. But there are seven matters concerning which special care must be expended to ensure just proportion: (1) equilibrium of temperament; (2) selection of the articles of food and drink; (3) evacuation of effete matters; (4) safeguarding the composite; (5) maintaining the purity of the air respired; (6) guarding against extraneous contingencies; and (7) moderation in regard to the movements of the body and the motions of the mind, with which may be included sleep and wakefulness.

From all these considerations you will now perceive that there is no single fixed limit to which equilibrium or health is to be assigned. None of the temperaments enters into it. Health and equilibrium vary (in range) from time to time. That is to say, it is a state comprised—within two limits.

On Diagnosis Signs and Symptoms

1.1. Introduction

Signs and symptoms indicate the present, past and future states of the three states of the body (health, illness, neutrality). According to Galen, knowledge of the present state is of advantage only to the patient as it helps him to follow the proper course of management. Knowledge of the past state is useful only to the physician inasmuch as its disclosure by him to the patient brings him a greater respect for his professional advice. Knowledge of the future state is useful to both. It gives an opportunity to the patient to be forewarned to adopt necessary preventive measures and it enhances the reputation of the physician by correctly forecasting the future developments.[1]

The signs belonging to the first category are called "demonstrative." Those of the second category are "commemorative." Those of the third are named "prognostic."

The signs of health include: (1) those which denote an equable temperament; and (2) those which denote equability of the composite: (i) substantial (creaturely form, position, quantity, number); (ii) accidental (comeliness, beauty); and (iii) final (fulfilling functions and fulfilled function).

Every organ is healthy whose functions are adequately performed. The functional efficiency of the principal organs may be assessed by observing, in the case of the brain, voluntary movements, sensory activity and mental functions; in the case of the heart, the condition of the pulse and respiration; and in the case of the liver, stools and urine. If the stools and urine are of a meat juice color, there is likely to be inefficiency of the liver.

Some signs of disease are pathognomonic of disease. Thus, rapid pulse-rate in fever itself indicates fever. Other signs indicate the position of the disease. Thus a hard pulse denotes diaphragmatic pleurisy. Undulant pulse denotes inflammation in the substance of the lung. Other signs indicate the cause of the disease. For instance, the signs of plethora or of depraved states in their various forms.

Sometimes the signs and symptoms may continue throughout the illness, i.e., persistence of acute fever, piercing pain, dyspnea, dry cough and serrete pulse—essential to pleurisy. In some cases, the signs and symptoms may however appear only at a particular stage of the illness or the signs may appear towards the end of an illness, like the signs of crisis, signs indicating maturation or lack of maturation and signs portending death. These symptoms are often associated rather with acute illnesses.

Sometimes other symptoms concern the state of the members. Some of them are discernible by the special senses—color, hardness, softness, heat, cold and the like. Others are discernible by all senses together—the form of the member, its position (posture, attitude), its size, its movements, or stillness. Some symptoms point to an interior state as when tremor of the lower lip reveals nausea. Changes in measure and number reveal internal states. For instance, shortness of fingers denotes small liver.

Sometimes morbid states are discernible by the special senses. Thus a black or yellow color of the excrement reveals a morbid state. Black or yellow jaundice of the whole body reveals an obstruction in the biliary passages.

Sometimes states are manifested to the sense of hearing—eructations reveal gastrectasis and defective digestive power.

Sometimes odors and tastes also enable one to become cognizant of morbid states.

Sometimes other visible evidences: curved nails denote ulceration in the bronchi, phthisis, and "hectic."

Signs and symptoms based on rest and movement are of special importance (gestures, postures, attitudes). The states of the body are revealed by its movements or absence of movement: (1) motionlessness of the body as a whole: in apoplexy, epilepsy (coma), syncope, palsy; or (2) unusual movements: shivering, tremor, twitching, sneezing, yawning, stretching, cough, trembling, spasms (especially note in which member this begins).

Some of these unusual movements are: (1) physiological (hiccup); (2) while others are symptomatic (convulsion or spasm, tremor); (3) and some are voluntary (tossing about in bed and turning from side to side); (4) others are partly voluntary, partly involuntary (cough, micturition, defecation). In some of these the voluntary is overruled by the involuntary (cough), while in others the voluntary overrules the involuntary (micturition and defecation, occurring too slowly owing to interference by the will); and (5) involuntary movements: some of these are evident to the senses (shivering), others are not (quivering, jactitation).

These movements vary: (1) in regard to their nature: thus, cough is intrinsically more energetic and powerful than quivering; and (2) in extent—thus the act of sneezing entails the use of more muscles than the act of coughing does. Coughing is accomplished simply by the movements of the chest, sneezing entails movements of the head as well as of the chest; in degree of associated mental anxiety. Dry hiccup is associated with a greater degree of mental anxiety than the movement of coughing although the latter is more vigorous, being reinforced by the natural instinctive drive. In some cases the movement is aided by an essential primary instrument. Thus, defecation is aided by the abdominal muscles. In other cases the aid is extraneous. Thus, the natural act of coughing may be aided by the atmosphere; in origin: these movements vary: (1) according to the member—cough, nausea; (2) according to the instinctive drives involved—jactitation originates in the vegetative drives while the act of coughing originates in the sensitive drives; (3) according to the humour concerned—thus cough proceeds from an excretion while twitching from a gaseous agent. These are all evidences of conditions in the members and are chiefly external in character. Some of them reveal internal conditions as, for instance, redness of the cheeks is a sign of pulmonary inflammation.

There are also internal evidences of external conditions and to discern these a perfect anatomical knowledge is necessary.

1.2. The Signs of Internal Disease

It is necessary for the diagnosis of internal disease that one should have knowledge of the anatomy of various organs. Thus, one must know about: (1) The essential structure of each member, whether fleshy or not; what its normal form is. One must know (i) whether the swelling, for instance, is according to the proper form of the member or not; (ii) whether it is proportioned or not; (iii) whether it is possible for anything to be retained within the given member or not; (iv) whether that which is within (for example jejunum) can escape; (v) whether there can be retention in and also escape from the member; (vi) what the material is which can be retained in it or discharged from it. (2) Its site: from this one judges whether pain or swelling is actually in the part or at some distance from it. (3) Its relations: by this knowledge one judges whether pain is arising per se or reflexly from the surroundings or whether the matter is an inflammatory mass arose in it or has entered into it from neighboring parts. If it be a "superfluity which escapes, is this the matter itself or is the affected member merely the channel by which the matter finds egress from the body? (4) How to decide wither the discharge could have come from the supposedly affected member or not. (5) The normal function of a member—from interference with function one recognizes the diseased state.

This is the purpose of the study of anatomy. A knowledge of anatomy is also necessary to enable the doctor to control diseases involving the interior organs.

The study of the significance of the symptoms of internal diseases should follow the following six headings: (1) Interference with function. The functions have already been described in regard to their qualities and degrees. The indications here are primary and constant; (2) Discharges: the indications here are constant, but not primary. They (1 and 2) are constant in that they are always associated with morbid states. They are not primary because they denote maturation or interference with maturation. Those that are neither primary nor constant are: (3) pain; (4) swelling; (5) altered position; and (6) special symptoms.

1.2.1. Interference with Function

When a function does not proceed normally, it shows that the agent at work is attacking the instinctive drive itself and the loss of function is secondary to disease of the organ subserving that function. There are three ways in which function is interfered with: (1) impairment such as failing eyesight, near sight, digestion impaired in rate or degree; (2) alteration—as when the eye sees that which is not there or perceives incorrectly; when the stomach digests food wrongly and causes it to decompose; (3) destruction—as when there is entire loss of vision; or entire loss of digestive power.

1.2.2. Significance of Discharges and Retentions

The significance of discharges and retentions include: (1) Retention of that which is normally discharged (e.g., retention of urine or feces); (2) Abnormal discharge: (i) from the substance of a member (a) itself diagnostic (for example, when a piece of cartilaginous tissue is coughed up, this is a proof of deep ulceration in the air-passages); (b) diagnostic by reason of its dimensions or amount (passage of flakes in dysentery—if they are large flakes, the ulcer is in the large intestine; if fine, the ulceration is in the small intestine); (c) color of the discharge (if urinary sediment is red, it shows the disease is in the fleshy organs such as the kidney; if white it shows the disease is in a muscular organ like the bladder); (ii) Not from the substance of a member: (a) entirely unnatural (thus healthy humours or blood should not be discharged at all); (b) abnormal in quality (thus depraved blood may be discharged physiologically, or not); (c) abnormal in substance (calculus); (d) abnormal in quantity (polyuria, oliguria, excess of fecal discharge, paucity of feces which is either abnormal in quality like black feces, black urine or discharge by unsuitable or unnatural channels: i.e., passage of faces by the mouth in cases of strangulated hernia).

1.2.3. The Significance of Pain

The significance of pain includes: (a) its site—if right-sided, examine the liver; if left-sided, the spleen; and (b) its type, which reveals its cause. Severe pain indicates inflammation in a non-essential member, or in a member which has lost sensation, but has become greatly distended by foreign matter. Incisive pain shows that the diseased material is sharp, acid or acrid.

1.2.4. The Significance in Regard to Inflammations

The significance in regard to inflammations include: (1) as to essence —erysipelatous inflammation denotes bilious humour; scirrhus (induration) denotes atrabilious humour; (2) as to position—whether on (liver or spleen) the right side or the left; and (3) as to shape—a moon-shaped swelling in the right hypochondrium points to the liver; an elongated swelling refers one to the overlying muscles (rectus and adnexa).

1.2.5. The Significance of Site and Relations

The significance of site and relations includes: the site may be self-evident. The relations vary in significance according to the morbidic agent. Thus a lesion in the fingers may result from injury to the brachial plexus in the neck.

1.2.6. The Significance of Special Symptoms

The significance of special symptom include: wasting; black tongue; and burning fever.[2]

1.3. The Distinction Between the Disease in Itself and Its Secondary Effects

Diseases may affect a member primarily or only secondarily. Thus, a disease of the stomach may become associated with one in the head. It is necessary to distinguish between the two conditions as being respectively primary and secondary. To do this, note which arises first, and then note which of the two morbid conditions persists. The former is judged to be primary; the one which develops later is considered to be secondary. Conversely, the disease is secondary which comes after the first, and ceases when the first is relieved.

Errors may arise, however, because a primary disease may escape the senses (being painless) at first, and its effect may not become manifest until after the secondary disease has appeared and so one is liable to regard the secondary ones as primary, and overlook the real root of the disease.

To guard against this mistake, the physician must know the anatomical interrelations of the members, and also the several affections which each member may show. Some of these are evident to our senses, others are not. He must also avoid giving a definite diagnosis of the root of the disease until he has had time to consider the possibility of some of the states being secondary or not.

Therefore the physician will diligently question the patient in order to discover signs indicative of the various affections which can possibly occur secondarily in the neighboring or related organs. If these are not painful (tender), the patient is unaware of them, and the various signs and symptoms may be only distantly related in his mind. He cannot know the relation between remote symptoms and the real root of the disease. The wisdom of the physician alone can determine this.

It is easier if one recalls the various points to memory under the heading of hindrances to function. If these are prior in time, the malady is secondary.

Some affections of members are usually secondary to others. Thus, an affection of the head is usually secondary to one or other of the morbid states of the stomach. The converse is only very rarely true. All the signs of the primary and secondary temperaments will be set forth in a general way now, leaving the signs of each special organ to its appropriate place. The visible signs of a composite disease are detected by the senses, but the internal symptoms of the body as a whole cannot be described in a general way except with difficulty—with the exception of the signs of plethora, of obstructions in passages, of inflammatory masses, and of loss of continuity. It is best to describe all these together when we describe them under their specific organs.

1.4. The Diagnostic Signs of the Temperaments

The signs from which the variety of the temperament is discernible can be arranged under ten groups: (1) the feel of the patient; (2) the state of the muscles, flesh and fat; (3) the hair; (4) the color of the body; (5) the form of the members; (6) the rapidity with which members respond to heat and cold; (7) signs derived from sleep and wakefulness; (8) signs derived from the state of the functions; (9) signs derived from the expulsive drive and from the quality of discharges; and (10) signs derived from the states of the mind during action and passion.

1.4.1. The Feel of the Patient

One notes whether the feel of the patient corresponds to health in temperate climes and temperate atmosphere by means of touch. If it corresponds, the temperament is equable. If the physician is himself healthy in temperament and finds the patient cold or hot, softer or harder or rougher than normal, and this is not to be explained by the state of the atmosphere or of a previous cold water bath or some other contingency rendering the body soft or rough, though normal he then knows the finding is due to an intemperament.

The state of the fingernails should be noticed. Softness or dryness of the nails not due to an extraneous agent, informs one of the state of the temperament. These qualities are not in themselves a sufficient criterion. There must be signs of balance between heat and cold. For (a) heat, by its resolving it effect, would modify hardness and roughness of feel, and make the patient seem to be attempered and his nature seem soft and moist. Or, (b) cold—i.e. the opposite—by reason of the great congelation and inspissation it induces, would make the softness of feel in an attempered person seem hard, and give the impression that his nature was dry. For instance, take snow and the sun. Snow congeals and causes coagulation; the sun causes aggregation of particles. Many persons with a cold temperament are soft to the feel, and also spare in habit owing to the presence of much immaturity in them.

1.4.2. The State of the Muscles, Flesh and Fat

Plentiful muscular development denotes moist temperament, and warm temperament if the muscles are firm. Scanty muscular development with very little fat shows that the temperament is dry. Oiliness and fat always denote cold temperament, and the muscles are then also flabby.

If at the same time there is constriction of the veins and lack of blood, and if there is weakness from lack of food (because there is too little blood to enable it to furnish the requirements of the tissues), this shows that this temperament is inborn and habitual. But if these other signs are absent, it shows the temperament to be an acquired one.

Lessening of the amount of oil and fat in the subcutaneous tissues always indicates a hot temperament, because the substance of oil and fat is the oiliness of the blood, and that is derived from colds Hence these things are less plentiful in the liver-region, and more plentiful over the intestines. There is not more oil and fat over the heart than over the liver, except as to matter; it is not temperament or "form" which accounts for this; it is simply that the "nature" of the heart depends for its maintenance on the presence of such-like "matter."

Congelation of oil and fat over the body is greater or less according as the heat is more or less in degree.

If the body is fleshy, and the amount of fat and oil not great, the temperament is hot and moist.

If the body is very muscular, and there is much oil, but little fat, this denotes excessively humid temperament. If extremely fleshy, this denotes superfluity of moisture and cold. It is evidence that the body has become cold and moist.

The more spare the body is in habit, the more likely is it to be cold and dry; or (less likely) hot and dry; or, dry, for such a body is attempered as to heat and cold. Or, hot, because such a body is attempered as to moisture and dryness.

1.4.3. The Hair

The points to note are: (a) rate of growth; (b) amount; (c) fineness or coarseness of texture; (d) straightness or curliness; (e) color.

1.4.3.1. Rate of Hair Growth

Rate of growth: slow growth, or absence of growth, without evidence of lack of blood denotes extremely humid temperament. More rapid growth denotes a less humid temperament, rather tending to dryness. (Heat and coldness of temperament are shown by other signs given above than the hair.)

1.4.3.2. Amount of Hair

Amount: if the temperament is both hot and dry, the hair grows much more rapidly, and each hair is numerous and coarse. Abundance of hair means heat, while coarseness indicates much fumosity. Therefore, the hair is more plentiful in adolescent persons than in puberty, as the humours of the latter are vaporose, not fumose. The opposite characters denote the respective contraries.

1.4.3.3. Form of the Hair

Form of the hair: curly hair denotes hot and dry temperament. It may be that there is tortuosity of the minute channels and pores, and this cannot change even if the temperament changes. But the two primary causes would change if the temperament changed. Straight hair denotes cold and temperament.

1.4.3.4. Color of the Hair

Black hair indicates hot temperament. In such cases oxidative processes are in excess of the mean. Brown hair indicates cold temperament. Tawny and red hair indicates equable temperament. There is an excess of unburned heat so that the hair always grows red. Therefore, there is a proneness to anger (a form of heat). Very fair hair indicates a cold and very moist temperament while grey hair indicates a cold and very dry one. Note how plants lose their dark or green color when dried and become grey or white. In the human being, this change is produced towards the close of drying or desiccant diseases.[3]

The cause of grey hair: Aristotle stated that hair turns grey because it takes on the color of the serous humour.[4] Galen ascribed it to a mustiness accompanying the nutriment supplied to the hair which retards its movement and penetration into the pores (of the hair) (i.e. hair-sac). As a matter of fact, there is little difference between the two views, because the whiteness of the serous humour is physically due to the same cause as the whiteness of the mustiness. The subject really belongs to physics.

Observation also shows that atmosphere and geographical situation affects the hair. One would not expect to find the hair red (which denotes equable temperament) in a black person even though his temperament were equable; nor would one expect to find black hair (which denotes hot temperament) in a Slav, even though his temperament were hot.

1.4.3.5. Relation of Character of the Hair to Age

In puberty the hair is as in northern countries; in youth, as in southerly countries; after the age of fifty it is between the two. Abundance of the hair at puberty reveals the future temperament. As the person grows, it precedes the formation of atrabilious humour, and in the elderly person it shows that atrabilious humour is actually present.

1.4.4. The Color of the Body

Pallor indicates a cold temperament and the accompanying feature is lack of blood. Yellowish color indicates a hot temperament which is accompanied by lack of blood, and increase of bilious humour. Ruddiness indicates a hot temperament with abundance of blood, sanguine or bilious temperament. Sub-ruddiness indicates a hot temperament with dominance of bilious humour. Occasionally it denotes lack of blood, provided there is no bilious humour present in the blood as is the case in convalescence. A dark brown body indicates an extremely cold temperament. This is because sanguineous humour is dominant and there is deficient coagulability of the blood and it darkens and alters the color of the skin at the same time. A brown colored body indicates a hot temperament. A body the color of eggplant indicates a cold and dry temperament. The heat is such as follows upon pure atrabilious humour. A chalky body indicates a cold temperament where the serous humour is in excess. A leaden colored body indicates a cold and moist temperament. The atrabilious humour is only slightly in excess. This is because there is a trace of green in the whiteness. The latter depends on the serous humour and moistness of temperament. The greenness depends on congelative change in the blood because this tends to a blackness which, mingled with serous humour, produces a greenish tint. A grey and white body indicates a cold temperament. An ivory white body indicates a cold temperament where serous humour is in excess and the choleric humour is scanty.[5]

1.4.4.1. The Color of the Eyes

It is not easy, but it is possible, to assess the temperament of the brain from the color of the eyes.

1.4.4.2. Changes of Color

A change to yellow (yellowish-white): suspect disorder of the liver; change to yellowish-black: suspect disorder of the spleen; change to yellowish-green: suspect piles (this does not always hold good (marginal reading). These suggestions only apply for the moment when the change of color takes place.

1.4.4.3. The Color of the Tongue

It is not easy to assess the temperament of the stomach, intestines and veins from the color of the tongue, any more than it is to assess the temperament of the brain from the color of the eyes. There may be two different colors simultaneously in two members as a consequence of a disease. Thus, the tongue may become white and the countenance dusky. This occurs in jaundice when this is due to an intense acridity of the bilious humour.

1.4.5. The Form of the Members

1.4.5.1. Hot Temperament

Indication from members as to hot temperament include: big broad chest; large limbs; no narrowing or shortening of the hands or feet;

conspicuous full veins; big strong pulse; the muscles round the joints large (for growth and the form of composite structures requires heat).

1.4.5.2. Cold Temperament

Indication from members as to cold temperament include: the contraries of all the above. The natural drives and the formative drive are impaired by cold, so that the natural-functions are not perfectly carried out.

1.4.5.3. Dry Temperament

Indication from the members as to dry temperament include: roughness, curvature of form; joints conspicuous. Adam's apple prominent. Nasal cartilage conspicuous; nose of medium size.

1.4.5.4. Moist Temperament

Indication from the members as to moist temperament include: the contraries.[6]

1.4.6. The Rapidity With Which Organs Respond to Heat and Cold

If a member becomes "hot" rapidly and easily, it shows that it is hot in temperament, because change in the direction of its own temperament is more readily undergone than in the opposite direction. Similarly, if the organ behaves in the contrary way, it will be of cold temperament.

Some assert that it is otherwise, because we know they say that a thing only reacts to its contrary and not to its like. But if that were the case, it would follow that a thing would react more strongly to its like. But the reply to this is that two things are only really alike when one does not interact with the other; we then know that their respective qualities are of like "species" and "nature."

Of two things A and B, if B is less hot than A, we cannot speak of its being "like A." As long as one of the two is hotter, they cannot be called "alike." One is cold compared with the other. So an interaction (on the part of the body) is possible. B would be cold compared with A, not hot. B, too, may react with something else which is colder than itself [say C] besides reacting with "cold" [say D]. C or D may enhance the intrinsic quality of B according as they are stronger than B or not. It is easier for it to change towards that which enhances this quality of B or neutralizes the opposite quality of B on condition that the new causative agent harmonizes with A and B and neutralizes the temperamental nature.

Therefore it is clear that when the nature is of hot temperament heat will not show any action on it until the influence of the contrary cold has first been removed, and this is achieved by preventing the malefaction (which tends to be produced by a hot temperament) from becoming greater. The result is that if both events occur simultaneously, and the inhibiting agent is destroyed, they will mutually help one another in producing heat, and the two qualities will thus reach an acme.

When the body is exposed to foreign heat, however, the balance of temperament is likely to be destroyed. The innate heat of the body is all-important for resisting this. We depend on our innate heat for the neutralization of "hot" poisons, and for their expulsion and for the dissolution of their substance.

Innate heat, therefore, is the instrument of human nature for combating the injurious action of extraneous or foreign heat. By its means, the breath gets rid of it, expels it, disperses it, and oxidizes its material basis. Further, it combats the injurious action of foreign "cold," expelling it "by contrary." Coldness has not this power. It is only the contrary to coldness i.e. foreign heat—which can combat or repress it. Coldness cannot combat extraneous "cold." Innate heat does.

Innate heat is that which protects the natural humours from being overruled by foreign calorific agents. If the innate heat is strong, the natural drives are able to work through it, upon the humours, and so effect digestion and maturation, and so maintain them within the confines of the healthy state. The humours move according to its ministration. Extraneous or foreign "heat" cannot interfere with this movement, and so they do not undergo putrefactive decomposition. If the ingrate agent is feeble, the natural drives are harassed in the regulation of the humours. For the instrument the intermediary between the natural drives and the humours is enfeebled. Stagnation sets in and foreign heat now finds the humours no longer opposed to its action. It overcomes them. It utilizes them in its own way, and imparts a foreign movement to them; and the result is what is known as "putrefaction."

Therefore, it is clear that the innate heat is the instrument of all the faculties, whereas coldness can only help them secondarily. That is why one speaks of "innate heat," but not of "innate cold;" and why that which is proportionate to heat is not comparable with cold.[7]

1.4.7. The Signs Derived from Sleep and Wakefulness

The sensitive drives make use of these things frequently, in a manner corresponding to the primary qualities. Thus we say that in the wakeful state the body is the instrument of the soul.

If there is equipoise between sleep and wakefulness, it means that the temperament (especially of the brain) is equable. If sleep dominates, it denotes a cold and moist temperament (of the brain), whereas if wakefulness dominates, it shows a dry and hot temperament (especially in the brain).[8]

1.4.8. The Signs Derived from the State of the Functions

Functions[9] may be weakened, exalted, depraved, obstructed in their action, or abolished.

Equable temperament: the activities of the body proceed fully and perfectly and naturally

Hot temperament: there is over-activity, exaggerated activity; rapid growth of stature; increased rate of growth of hair; early eruption of the teeth.

Cold temperament: the activities lessen and become sluggish and delayed, but a hot temperament may cause weak and sluggish activity only if a deviation from the natural course is associated with weakness.

Many natural functions may slow down or lessen owing to heat. Thus, in the case of sleep, sometimes there is insomnia or lack of sleep from the effect of the heat of a hot temperament. Similarly some of the natural states may be intensified by cold. Thus, again, in the case of sleep, though this is not strictly the outcome of natural functions, but only an effect conditional upon some causal agent, because the necessity for sleep for life and health is not absolute. It enables the breath to separate off from its impeding factors the fatigue-substances. There is need for a recumbent posture after a meal. One cannot achieve two (contrary) things at the same time. Hence the need for sleep is simply some impotency. It is not included in "natural necessity." And if its exclusion be "natural" in the sense that it is inevitable, this is only because the word "natural" is here used for "the inevitable." One word is being made stand for two things. But the most accurate application of the term is to "equable temperament," for it is this upon which equability of functions and their final completion depends. To use the term in regard to the four qualities—heat, coldness dryness, moisture is only hypothetical.

Among the "strong" ("*jalal*") actions which denote a hot temperament are: a powerful voice; a harsh or coarse voice; a rapid way of talking; constantly talking; anger; rapid gestures; and blinking of the eyelids. Before deducing a hot temperament from these, one must make sure there is no local cause for them, and that they are not confined to one particular member.

1.4.9. The Signs Derived from the Expulsive Drive and from the Quality of Discharges

The temperament is hot if the waste matters are retained and if the feces, urine, sweat, etc., are strong in odor, acrid, of normal color, and show the normal degree of oxidation and maceration in the case of matters which normally undergo such changes. If the signs are contrary, the temperament is cold.[10]

1.4.10. The Signs Derived from the States of the Mind During Action and Passion

Cold temperaments show the opposites to those given for hot temperaments; moist, the opposites to those given for dry. This and most of the above refers to the congenital or innate temperament. Now we refer to acquired temperaments ("intemperaments").[11]

1.5. Evidences of the Four Primary Intemperaments

The signs of a morbid state to which there is a tendency to an acquired hot temperament is indicated when inflammatory conditions become febrile and there is a loss of vigor of a cold acquired temperament or intemperament when fevers are related to the serous humour and rheumatism develops, and of a moist or dry intemperament when there is lassitude.

Evidence of the functional power indicates deficient energy with a hot intemperament, deficient digestive power with a cold intemperament, difficult digestion with a moist or dry intemperament. Subjective sensations indicate a bitter taste in the mouth, excessive thirst, and a sense of burning at the cardiac orifice with hot intemperament; a lack of desire for fluids with a cold intemperament; mucoid salivation and sleepiness with a moist intemperament and insomnia and wakefulness with a dry intemperament.

Physical signs of a hot intemperament are indicated by a pulse extremely quick and frequent while approaching the weak type met with in lassitude; a cold intemperament is indicated by flaccid joints; a moist intemperament is indicated by diarrhea and swollen eyelids; a dry intemperament is indicated by rough skin and spare habit which is acquired and not inborn.

In regard to foods and medicines with a hot intemperament, calefacients are all harmful while infrigidants benefit; with a cold intemperament infrigidants are all harmful while calefacients benefit; with a moist intemperament, moist articles of diet are harmful; with a dry intemperament, dry regime is harmful while humectants benefit (hot water, rarefied oils are beneficial to the dry temperament and are avidly taken up).

In relation to weather, a hot intemperament is worse in the summer and a cold intemperament is worse in the winter. A dry intemperament is bad in the autumn.

1.6. The Signs of a Harmonious Temperament: Symmetry, Beauty of Form, and Good Conformation

In addition to the signs of normal temperament already given, there are: (a) To the feel, the body imparts sensations mean between hotness, coldness, dryness, moisture, softness, hardness. (b) In color, the body shows a balance between whiteness and redness. (c) In build, the body is neither bulky nor spare although on the whole inclined to be bulky. (d) The veins of the skin are neither prominent nor submerged; they are separated and spread. (e) The hair is neither profuse nor sparse, thick nor thin, curly nor straight, black nor white. During puberty they tend to a tawny shade rather than black, in youth they tend to blackness. Full hair where hair should be. (f) The person is equally inclined for sleep and for wakefulness.[12] (g) The person has agreeable dreams arousing hopefulness, with fragrant perfumes and alluring voices, visions and agreeable companionship. (h) Mental faculties include: vigor of imagination, intellectual power, and memory. Emotions are balanced between excess and deficiency, for example, between courage and timidity, between anger and patience, between sternness and clemency, between vacillation and perseverance. (i) Perfection in all functions.[13]

A person with such a temperament will have a happy expression, will be lovable and contented, moderate in desire for food and drink, possessing a good gastric digestion, good hermetic alley venous digestion, and good alternative and assimilative flower all through the tissues. The waste matters will be moderate in amount and will be discharged through the proper channels.

1.7. The Indications Afforded by Congenital Abnormalities: Asymmetry, Misproportion, Unshapeliness, and Ugliness

In brief, there is non-uniformity of temperament among the members; or, perchance, the principal members depart from equability and come to be of contrary temperament, one deviating towards one, another to its contrary. If the components of the body are out of proportion, it is unfortunate both for talent and reasoning power. Thus,

(1) a tall person with a large abdomen and short face and round head, and short fingers; (2) a person of small stature, with small head, much flesh in the face and forehead, and even in the neck and feet—the face like the full moon, the jaws rounded and massive. Similarly, (3) if the head and forehead were round but the face very round (long, marginal reading), and the neck very thick, and if the eyes are sluggish in movement. Such persons would be the very last of people to be classed as in good health.

1.8. The Signs of Plethora

Humoural changes may be quantitative or qualitative. Regarding plethora there are these same two aspects. Plethora in regard to cavities, tubes and juice canals (quantitative) and plethora in regard to power or strength (vitality; qualitative),

1.8.1. Quantitative Plethora

In quantitative plethora (plethora of the channels of the body), humours and vital force are of normal quality but so excessive in quantity that the vessels become distended. In these cases exertion is apt to cause rupture of blood vessels with the humours blocking the "passages" thus causing choking of throat, epilepsy and apoplexy. This type of plethora needs treatment by venesection.

1.8.2. Qualitative Plethora

In the case of qualitative plethora (plethora of strength of instinctive drives), the error is not in quantity of humours but in unhealthiness of quality whereby the instinctive drives are embarrassed and they become inefficient for the processes of digestion and maturation. A person who is in this state is in danger of putrefactive disorders.

1.8.3. Plethora in General

Speaking in general of the signs of plethora of the first type are either objective or subjective. Objective: red face; full of veins; tightness of skin; sluggish movements or gestures; full pulse, high-colored urine; dense urine; scanty appetite. Subjective: sense of weight in the limbs, weak vision; dreams in which there is a sense of weight—as when one dreams one is unable to move or is carrying a heavy weight or cannot give utterance to words. This kind of dream may be compared with that associated with attenuation of humours or where the humours are moderate in amount for here one dreams one is flying through the air or moving at a great speed.[14]

1.8.4. The Signs of Plethora with the Faculties or Drives

The signs of plethora in respect of the instinctive drives are heaviness, sluggishness, loss of appetite (these are also present in the preceding type), disinclination for exertion, and sense of burdensomeness.

If the plethora of the instinctive drive is unaccompanied by plethora of humours, the veins are not as distended and the skin is not as tense or the pulse as full and large or the urine as gross (dense) or as red in color. There is no lassitude except after undue movement and exercise and activity. The dreams consist of sensations of itching, stinging, burning, and of fetid odors. However, in the case of plethora of the instinctive drives, illness ensues before all its signs are manifest.

1.8.5. Additional Remarks

The age of the patient gives a clue to the kind of humour likely to be dominant. Excess of sanguineous humour is shown by signs akin to those of plethora and some of the signs given are accounted for by simple plethora. When the atrabilious humour is in excess, the blood is dusky and heavier than normal. Atrabilious humour is seldom in excess in pale and slight persons.[15]

1.9. The Signs of the Dominant Humour

1.9.1. Blood

The signs of predominance of blood[16] resemble those of quantitative plethora and are characterized by feelings of heaviness in the body, especially behind the eyes, over the head and across the temples. Stretching and yawning is frequent. There is a tendency to excessive sleep and the mind gets dull. Such persons are easily tired and often complain of a sweet taste in the mouth and usually have a red tongue. They are also predisposed to frequent appearance of boils over the body and ulcers on the tongue. Bleeding from the gums, nostrils and piles is frequent. Occasionally, the excess of blood can be recognized from the temperament of the person, his age, residence, previous habits and treatments and the characteristic dreams of seeing excessive blood or red things i.e., sight of a large quantity of blood being lost or someone being soaked in blood or some other such vision.

1.9.2. Phlegm

The signs of phlegm are excessive pallor, flabbiness of the body, cold and moist skin, excessive salivation and viscidity of the saliva. There is diminution of thirst, especially in the elderly, and particularly so when the phlegm is sour. A weak digestion with acid eructations, pale urine, excessive sleepiness, flabbiness of the muscles, mental torpor and softness of the pulse with slow rate and speed are characteristics of this condition. Age, occupation, residence, previous history and treatment are also helpful in identifying the predominance of phlegm. Dreams of water, canals, cold, ice, rain and thundering hail storms denote phlegm.

1.9.3. Yellow Bile (Choler)

Yellow color of the eyes and complexion, bitter taste in the mouth, rough and dry tongue and dryness of the nostrils are typical signs of yellow bile. Cool breezes are generally comforting. Excessive thirst, rapidity of pulse, lack of appetite are signs. Nausea with bilious vomiting of green or yellowish color, irritative diarrhea and often tingling of the skin are signs which point to the predominance of yellow bile. Temperament, age, occupation, residence, climate, previous habits and past treatments also help in the diagnosis. Characteristic dreams are of flames of fire and flags of yellow color. Additional signs of the yellow bile are that things seem yellow and there is burning and irritation after hot baths and on exposure to the sun.

1.9.4. Black Bile (Melancholy)

The characteristic signs of this condition are dry and dark skin, thick and dark blood, presence of anxiety, burning in the epigastrium, false appetite, turbid urine of a blue, dark or red color, dark complexion and excessive hair. If the complexion is pale and the hair scanty, there is seldom any excess of black bile. Patches of pigmentation, chronic indolent ulcers and diseases of the spleen also indicate excess of black bile. Age, temperament, habits, residence, occupation and history of previous treatments are also helpful in the diagnosis. Dreams are usually full of anxiety and often of dark places, dark trenches and dark fearful objects.

1.10. The Signs of Stasis or Obstructions

Obstruction is due to the retention of some normal secretion with feelings of tension and other vague signs of plethora. The obstruction of a duct which is normally free and has a regular flow of some excretion produces a feeling of heaviness, i.e., stasis or congestion in the liver, due to the blockage of the out-going hepatic veins which produce abnormal accumulation of the material arriving from the intestine. This causes a feeling of weight and heaviness which is sometimes even more than what may be experienced in inflammation. Inflammation is differentiated from obstruction by the presence of fever and relative lack of heaviness and weight.

The blockage of a channel, which has a very little discharge, seldom causes heaviness; it is only the rupture of some blood vessel which produces this symptom. Obstruction of blood vessels produces pallor as in such cases the blood fails to reach the surface.[17]

1.11. The Signs of Gaseous Distension

There is pain and tenderness in the affected part from a loss of continuity and abnormal movements are frequently noted. There are also some characteristic sounds and a distinctive feel. The diagnosis of gas can be made from the following.

1.11.1. Pain

Gas produces tension, but instead of heaviness it actually feels light and tends to move from place to place. There is pain when the gas has produced loss of continuity in a sensitive organ. It does not produce pain in the bones and glandular tissues. When occasionally it is of a larger quantity it may produce painless fractures. If pain does occur it is generally due to the damage of some neighboring structure caught in between the broken ends of a bone.

1.11.2. Movement

Palpitation (of the heart) and twitchings (of muscles) indicate dispersion of gas by the affected organ.

1.11.3. Sound

This may be heard directly as in flatulence or indirectly by palpation as in the case of gas over the splenic region. Sound may also be studied by percussion as in the differentiation of tympanities from ascites.

1.11.4. Feel

Distension from gas (tympanities) can be differentiated from other swellings by the amount of its pressure required to overcome the tension. Gas does not produce any thrill like the collections of fluid and it also lacks the characteristic feel of a liquid material.

1.11.5. Distinctions

The difference between inflation and gaseous distension is not in substance but in form. The form or shape of the distended area is different when standing or lying down and manipulation will alter its position.

1.12. The Signs of Solid Swellings

The presence of external tumors is easily demonstrated to the sense of sight. Deeply placed inflammatory swellings are revealed by accompanying fever as well as by a sense of heaviness if the affected member be devoid of sensation or of stabbing pain as well as heaviness if the member be sentient. Interference or hindrance to function and movement of a part affords a further sign of the presence of a tumor. A certain degree of intumescence of the overlying part is a very important sign of an inflammatory mass if sensation has access to it. Cold swellings are not accompanied by pain.

It is difficult to describe the signs of tumors in a general manner. Even if one could do so it would be at the expense of wearisome words. That is why it is simpler to defer details to the special chapters. It will suffice for the present to say that wherever heaviness and not pain are perceived and the signs of dominance of the serous humour are present, this leaves no doubt about the swelling being of pituitous nature. If there are signs of dominance of the atrabilious humour, and the swelling is hard to the touch, it will be an atrabilious mass because induration is pre-eminent among the signs of this form of swelling.

Inflammatory swellings in nerves are extremely painful and fever is intense, there is an accelerated rhythm in stretching, causing the pain, and there is delirium. Swellings in any of the inward parts of the body cause the abdominal wall to become wasted. If they are inflammatory and undergo suppuration and track outward, they cause extremely severe pain with fever; the tongue becomes very rough and there is great wakefulness; the symptoms become more and more severe—notably the sense of heaviness and weight and stiffness in the affected part. Induration and tension become evident. Sudden emaciation of the body with hollowness of the eyes may develop.

But when the process of suppuration has attained maturity, fever is high, pain lessens, the pulse softens, throbbing subsides and itching replaces the pain. If there was much redness and induration, the redness lessens, and the induration is less noticeable. Pressure on neighboring organs lessen and all the causes of pain subside along with the great sense of heaviness. When finally the abscess bursts there is a rigor produced by the acridity of the sanious matter; fever increases again because of the movement and discharge of the pus; and the pulse becomes empty, unequal, weak, infrequent, small, broad and slow. There is loss of appetite; often the extremities grow warm.

The following signs after the bursting of an abscess are good: subsiding fever, easy breathing, return of strength, quick evacuation of pus through its proper channels.

Sometimes, however, with deep abscesses, pus passes from one member to another and this transference is sometimes beneficial, sometimes detrimental. It is beneficial when it passes from a principal organ to a subordinate one; as for instance, when it passes from the brain to the tissues behind the ears and from the liver to the groins. It is detrimental if it passes from an ignoble organ to a noble one or to a weaker or less resistant organ as for instance when pleurisy involves the heart or lung.

In the internal organs the inflammation may spread upwards or downward in a characteristic manner. If the spread is downward, there is a feeling of heaviness and tension across the lower abdomen and if it is upwards breathing becomes difficult and irregular and there is a sense of constriction in the chest with a sensation of burning and irritation rising upwards. Also there may be heaviness near the collar bone, headache and occasionally pain in the arm and the wrist. The spread of inflammation to the brain is a dangerous complication unless it localizes in the glands behind the ears. In these cases, as also in the inflammatory conditions of the abdomen, the occurrence of epistaxis is a favorable sign. A more comprehensive description of the abdominal inflammation will be given when the subject of inflammation is dealt with in the volume on diseases of the internal organs.

1.13. The Signs of Loss of Continuity

Loss of continuity in the external organs is easily recognized by inspection and palpation. In the internal organs the signs are: (a) pain of a throbbing, stabbing, or tearing nature, especially when there is no fever; (b) elimination of some humour, i.e., the expectoration of blood, or the discharge of this humour into a cavity or discharge of pus from some pre-existing inflammation or matured abscess. If the discharge is not from a matured inflammation it would relieve the heaviness and fever but would be otherwise followed by an aggravation of pain; (c) a complete or partial displacement of an organ, i.e., hernia or an intestinal obstruction.

Prognosis: As you are aware, both loss of continuity and the presence of (inflammatory swellings) are more grave when they occur in very sensitive fibromuscular members. In fact, such loss of continuity may prove fatal from syncope or spasm. The syncope is due to the violence of the pain; the spasms are due to the irritation of the nerves in which the parts are so rich. Next in severity comes loss of continuity near joints, because restoration can only be slow considering the undue mobility of the parts, and the fact that spaces are opened up in and round the joints, and matters readily flow into these spaces.

Endnotes
Introduction by Laleh Bakhtiar

1 Seyyed Hossein Nasr, *Three Muslim Sages*, pp. 23-24.
2 The Islamic medical tradition is the part of reference of this great textbook of Avicenna (Ibn Sina) which served to heal millions of people as this was the only medical textbook for 700 years in Europe alone. Translated into Latin, it served as the basis for Shakespere's psychology, among others. St. Thomas Aquinas has said: Anything Avicenna says is correct.
3 Nader Ardalan and Laleh Bakhtiar, *The Sense of Unity*, p. 11.
4 Ibid., p. 11.
5 Ibid., p. 13.
6 Ibid.,p. 13.
7 Ibid., p. 19.
8. R. A. Nicholson, *Rumi, Mystic and Poet*, p. 31.
9. Nader Ardalan and Laleh Bakhtiar, *op. cit.*, p. 19.
10 *Ibid.*, p. 19 which quotes S. H. Nasr, *Three Muslim Sages*, p. 112.
11 Seyyed Hossein Nasr, *Islamic Science: An Illustrated Study*, p. 161.
12 According to the Ayurvedic system, there are three bio-energies called *dosha (arkan)*. They are *vatha* [nervous spirit]: driving force. It relates mainly to the nervous system and the body's energy; *pitta* [animal spirit, fire] relates to digestion, metabolism, enzymes, acid and bile; *kapha* [natural spirit] relates to mucous membranes, phlegm, moisture, fat and lymphatics.

Seyyed Hossein Nasr points out: "It is worth drawing attention to the similarity between the words *ruh* and *rih* (the wind or air) in Arabic and to the Galenic doctrine that through the air breathed by the organism the life-force enters the body. It is also of significance to note that in Arabic as in many other languages the words for breath (*nafas*) and soul (*nafs*) are related. Therein lies a profound cosmological principle which is also related to the invocation of the Name of God (*dhikr*) as the central technique of Sufism for spiritual realization." *Sufi Essays*, p.27.
13 Seyyed Hossein Nasr, *Science and Civilization in Islam*, pp. 223-224.
14 Called *prana* or energy of life in the Ayurvedic system, it is comprised of energy which changes according to our circumstances, our diet, our lifestyles and the world around us. Some are positive and some are negative. We have to live in a way to attain energy balance. Energy controls the functions of every cell, thought, emotion, and action.

O.Cameron Gruner's Remarks

1 This was actually Gruner's conclusion, but because it explains the content of The Canon so well and because today we have grown so distant from Avicenna's concepts, we have placed it before Gruner's original introduction, which follows and expounds the differences between Avicenna and "modern medicine."
2 Altounyan, Lancet, I928, ii, 684.
3 St. Thomas Aquinas, *Summa Theologica*, p. 177.
4 See Introduction by O. Cameron Gruner, Doctrine of "the Constitution"
5 See notes to Avicenna *on Psychology*, Details Regarding the Emotions.
6 See Avicenna *on Diagnosis Signs and Symptoms*, Details Regarding Odor.
7 See Avicenna *on The Temperaments*, Details Regarding Age.
8 Notes to Avicenna *On the Four Temperamen*ts, Application of the Doctrine; notes to Avicenna *on Psychology*, Details Concerning Some of the Drives; List of Terms Applicable to Mental Faculties.
9 Notes to *On His Psychology*, List of Terms Applicable to Mental Faculties.
10 St. Thomas Aquinas, *Summa Theologica*, p. 203.
11 See Avicenna *on the Breath*.
12 For other cycles see Avicenna *on Illness*.
13 See Introduction by O. Cameron Gruner, Doctrine of "the Constitution."
14 Notes to Change in Vibration-rate.
15 Vallery-Radot, *Precis de Pathologie Medicale*.
16 *Uruj* (ascent), *nasul* (descent), *jalal* (majesty), *jamal* (beauty), *qada* (fate), *qadr* (destiny).
17 Cf. Bechold 112, Sckade 137, Pearson and Wyllie 160 and many other authorities.
18 See *On the Diagnosis of Signs and Symptoms*.
19 See *On the Diagnosis of The Pulse*.
20 See *On the Diagnosis of Signs and Symptoms*.
21 See *On Medicine and its Topics*.
22 Many other points are noted in Part Two.
23 See *On Treating Diseases, Disorders, Obstructions, Swellings and Managing Pain*.
24 M. O. Stanton, *An Encyclopedia of Face and Form Reading*.
25 Sir A. Garrod, *The Huxley Lecture on Diathesis*.
26 See *On the Classification of Types of Disease*.
27 St. Thomas Aquinas, *Summa Contra Gentiles*, ii, 75, p. 204.
28 *Ibid*., 205.
29 See Part Two.
30 F. Hartmann, *The Life of Paracelsus and the Substance of His Teachings*.
31 See Part Three.
32 J. Bauer, Int. Med., ii, 127.
33 The essay entitled "Progress," was Gruner's Appendix.
34 See Introduction by O. Cameron Gruner on knowledge.
35 See Part Four.
36 This is the beginning of Gruner's original Introduction.
37 *Les Grands philosophes*, p. 156.
38 Ameer Ali, *The Spirit of Islam*, p. 392.
39 For instance, at Cairo, established in 684 A.H. by the daughter of the Mameluke Sultan Malik Taher.

40 Ameer Ali, *The Spirit of Islam*, p. 392.
41 *Lehrbuch der Geschichte der Medizin*, i. 662.
42 *Arabian Medicine and Its Influence on the Middle Ages*, p. 57.
43 Ameer Ali, *ibid.*, p. 517.
44 Old saying quoted by Ameer Ali, ibid, p. 125.
45 *Many Days in Morocco*, pp. 32, 61.
46 Somerset Maugham, *On a Chinese Screen*.
47 Sir Henry Howarth, *History of the Mongols*.
48 Forke, T*he World-conception of the Chinese*.
49 Others include Brucell, Wilhelm, Ging, *Das Buch der Wardlungen aus dem chinesische*.
50 See Avicenna's *Introductory Words*.
51 See Avicenna's *Introductory Words*.
52 See *On Medicine and its Topics*.
53 See *On Medicine and its Topics*.
54 See *On Medicine and its Topics*.
55 *Ibid*.
56 See *On Medicine and its Topics*.
57 J. P. Bruce, *Chu Hsi: Philosophy of Human Natur*e, p. 168.
58 Chuang Tzu, Giles translation, p. 170.
59 *Ayurveda*, 1924, i, I.; and see also Weber, *History of Indian Literature*.
60 Forke, *Chinesische Mystik*, pp. 242, 243.
61 Lancet, 1927.
62 Cf. Forke, *ibid*.
63 Hume quoted by Maher, *Psychology*, p. 238.
64 Kempis, *Imitatio Christi*, ii, II.
65 St. Thomas, *Summa Contra Gentiles*, i, 53.
66 *Gulshan-i raz*, couplet 299, p. 30.
67 *Essays in Zen Buddhism*, p. 185.
68 *Ibid*., p. 200.
69 *Ibid*. p. 306.
70 *Rose Garden,* 1st ed., p. 120.
71 J. P. Bruce, *Chu Hsi: Philosophy of Human Nature*, i., 182.
72 The real authorship of the Libellus on the power of the hearts is disputed. Arnold of Villanova translated it into Latin (ca. 1235-1312).
73 Huineng, Susuki, *Essays in Zen Buddhism*, p. 203.
74 *Ibid*., p. 223.
75 *Kempis, Imitatio Christi*, i., 5.
76 St. Thomas Aquinas, *Summa Theologica*, Dominican translation.
77 Ibid., liv; lv. 2; lviii. 3,4; vol. 3, p. 51-87; Pegues, *Catechism of the Summa Theologica of St. Thomas Aquinas*, p. 18.
78 F. Hartmann, *The Life of Paracelsus*, p. 217.
79 Ed. Hughes, *Lancet*.
80 Sauvage, *Catholic Encyclopedia*, xii., 313.
81 Mercier, *Manuel of Modern Scholastic Philosophy*; Logique, 1904; de Wulf, *Catholic Encyclopedia*, xii., p. 26.
82 Maher, *Psychology*, p. 520.
83 Cf. Maher, *Psychology,* pp. 35, 36; and especially Wundt, *Catholic Encyclopedia,* xii., p. 35.

84 Maher, *Psychology*, p. 9.
85 In. Met. I., lect. 2.
86 *Summa Theologica*, II-III, q. 45, art. i.e.
87 *Ibid.*, ad. 2.
88 *Ibid.*, q. 9, a. 2, ad 3.
89 St. Thomas Aquinas, *Summa Contra Gentiles*.
90 *Ibid.*, ii. 3, I. p. 5.
91 *Catechism of the Council of Trent*, 1545-1563.
[Footnotes 92-110 not featured]
111 Wieger, p. 309 on Su-Wen.
112 See *On the Humours*.
113 See *On the Humours*.
114 See *On the Humours*.
115 See notes to *On Diseases, Causes and Symptoms*.
116 See *On Diagnosis, Signs and Symptoms*..
117 Ind. Med. Services.
118 *Ayurveda*, 1924, 2, i., 1.
119 Sontheimer, *Zusammengesetzte Heilmittel der Arabe*r, p. 91.
120 F. Hartmann, *Chinesische Heilmethoden*, Munch. Med. Woch., 1927; June 3rd, 935.
121 See *On Diagnosis of the Pulse*.
122 See *On Diagnosis of the Pulse*
123 The following paragraphs are interesting among many others.
124 *Arabian Medicine*, p. 34.
125 *Die Augenheilkunde des Ibn Sina*.
126 *Arabian Medicine and Its Influence on the Middle Ages*, p. 139.
127 E. G. Browne, *ibid.*, p. 26, 27.
128 *Manuel of Modern Scholastic Philosophy*.
129 Maher, *Psychology,* endnote, p. 31.
130 J. B. Bruce, *Chu Hsi and His Masters*, p. 137.

On Diagnosis Signs and Symptoms

1 The science of the diagnosis of disease by internal symptoms is founded upon six canons: (1) the patient's actions; (2) the waste of the body; (3) the nature of the pain; (4) the site of the pain; (5) swelling; (6) the effluvia given off by his person.

2 Joannitius gives a rather different classification of symptoms and signs, though summarizing from the same text. It may be said that every classification is a matter of personal convenience. There is not necessarily any principle involved, for the subject comprises so great a variety that a strictly logical classification serves no special purpose. In some cases symptoms are characteristic of a cause, in others of an error of function, in others of a special disease. To adhere consistently to one rule of classification necessarily entails the relegation of some symptoms which are important in actual practice to a subsidiary or insignificant position in the list. Therefore, it may be said that Avicenna's classification will hold good as well as any. The student obtains his knowledge from his own experience and not from memorizing a given list.

The following list of simple ailments or evidence of disease may be offered at this point: (1) Pain. the first evidence of disease or ill-health. Its localization is very significant and charts depicting its possible sites and their meaning are of great use. Thus headache is very commonly simply a sign of indigestion (gastric or intestinal) or constipation. The type of pain is most important. Thus pain in the abdomen relieved by pressure suggests gaseous distension due to abnormal fermentation of food whereas pain increased by pressure suggests inflammation. (2) Abnormal discharges. Abnormal in quantity (increased or diminished), such as diarrhea, polyuria. Abnormal in quality such as nose-bleeding, hemoptysis, expectoration, nasal discharge, salivation. Abnormal in manner, such as incontinence. (3) Abnormal acts. Vomiting, coughing, hiccup, eructations, yawning, sighing, shivering, sleepiness, insomnia, altered gait, altered posture (from palsy, exhaustion, collapse), tremors, twitchings, convulsions, etc. (4) Abnormal subjective sensations. In special senses: floating specks before the eyes in dyspepsia, ringing in the ears in cases of nervous debility, or after certain drugs or from wax; bitter taste in dyspepsia, dizziness arising from nerve derangement or circulatory errors. In general: nausea, palpitation, throbbing, labored breathing, altered appetite, thirst, sense of lassitude or asthenia, irritability, loss of memory. (5) Outward signs. Discolored or "heavy" eyes. Offensive breath in indigestion and constipation. Wasting or obesity. Hot and dry skin in fevers or states of mental excitement or from excess of salt in the diet. Cold sweating from exhaustion, etc. Altered color of skin. Edema of skin; skin-eruptions; signs derived from examination of the mouth. Pale tongue and gums from blood-deficiency, bleeding gums from excess of salt in diet and other causes; colored line on gums in metallic poisonings, coated tongue in digestive disturbances, loosened teeth from errors of diet or the use of adulterated foods, etc.

3 Color of the Hair

Color	*Corresponding Temperament*	*Remarks*
Black	Hot	In such cases oxidative processes are in excess of the mean (Joannitius).
Brown	Cold	
Tawny/Red	Equable	There is an excess of "unburned heat"so that the hair always grows red (Joannitius). Therefore the proneness to anger (a form of
Very Fair	Cold and very moist	Note how plants lose their dark or green color when dried and become white or red. In the human being, this change is produced towards the close of desiccant diseases.
Grey	Cold and very dry	

The following details are from Joannitius:

- Black: due to: smallness of crystalline lens; setting of the crystalline lens too far back; abundance of aqueous humour; turbidity thereof; uvea redundant; peculiarity of the visible "breath" (scanty or confused).
- Brown: due to the contraries of the above—crystalline lens large or further forward; paucity of albugineous humour; clearness of this; deficient quality of uvea; the visible breath plentiful or clear.
- Intermediate colors (black and brown mixed). The visible breath varies in amount and clarity.
- Grey: visible breath less plentiful.

4 Joannitius ascribed it to decomposition changes in the serous humour occurring in old age; greyness, he says, means excess of atrabilious humour.

5 See chart above.

6 Joannitius adds: fleshiness (excess of heat and moisture in the temperament); fatness (excess of moisture and intense coldness); leanness (hot temperament and intense dryness); delicate build: cold and very dry; massive build: cold and very moist or very cold and very moist; justness of form: well-balanced humours.

7 This passage is evidently an attempt to explain the nature of bacterial action and infection without the knowledge of the actual bacteria themselves. The description is so ingenious that it requires little change to modernize it. The following may be applied accordingly: (1) the meaning of innate heat; (2) the nature of "foreign heat" and "foreign cold"; (3) the meaning of the term "hot poison"; (4) the meaning of hot and cold as relative terms.

(1) Innate heat. This term, particularly in this passage, is equivalent to "vitality." This word describes a complex concept. Though regarded as vague and quite unsatisfactory today, it may be said to be amenable to reduction to a formula—and a formula into which several factors enter. The condemnation of the term is due to the non-recognition of this fact and non-recognition that many well-known and freely-accepted data belong to it.

(2) The nature of "foreign heat" and "foreign cold." These refer to material agents now known as pathogenic micro-organisms. The material substance which is stated by Avicenna to be oxidized by "innate heat," is the bacterial substance which as we know undergoes lysis in the course of the immunizing processes of the body. The "heat" refers to what we know as the bacterial toxins which act upon the thermogenic centers and produce numerous other effects on the tissues. The word "heat" thus comprises two things: the pyrexia produced by bacterial invasion may be theoretically distinguished from the innate heat, but practically speaking, the rise of temperature is generally admitted to be part of the so-called defensive mechanism against infections. The destruction of the bacteria, and of their products by anti-substances—these events are comprised in the words "dispersing the foreign heat." After all, both bacteria and products are "dispersed." We are only being told the same fact in different language.

In the case of foreign cold, here the organisms and products differ. But if the temperature becomes subnormal, the immunizing process is not ascribed to the lowered temperature. Recovery from the infection still depends on the "innate heat" or "vitality" that is, a series of processes of immunization which take place, whether the patient develops fever or not.

Avicenna considers that the formation of septic products is more likely if there is not much pyrexia on the ground that in such a case the bacteria, as we should say, meet with less resistance, and are enabled to produce those decompositions of the body fluids which we know to take place readily as soon as the vitality of a part is lowered.

(3) The meaning of the term "hot poisons." Clearly the word poison must be understood as covering both bacterial agents and their products. The toxic products may produce rise of temperature and are, therefore, reasonably called "hot." Others do not have this effect.

(4) The meaning of hot and cold as relative terms. In this passage a thing is hot or cold according to its effect on the bodily sensations or its effect on the heat centers of the body. Taken in its literal or surface meaning of hot temperature, cold temperature, the passage is of course pedantic and useless. It should be evident that the words "hot" and "cold" cannot possibly have meant literal heat and cold.

8 A strong inclination to sleep denotes debility—a loss of tone of the muscular power. Histologically, sleep depends on a break in the ideation-zone of the cerebral cortex. If there is a break in the layer below that, the sleep will be that of stupor or coma. The break in this situation is marked in amentia and dementia. Wakefulness or insomnia denotes poisons circulating n the blood, powerful sensory impulses (pain) or powerful emotions.

9 Functions may be weakened, exalted, depraved, obstructed in their action or abolished.

10 Signs Derived from the States of the Mind During Action and Passion

Evidence	*Name of Temperament*	*Corresponding*
Emotional Aspect	*Hot*	*Dry*
Concupscible	1. Shameless[1] 2. Excitable 3. Lively, vivacious	Infatuation: love, passion

Evidence	*Name of Temperament*	*Corresponding*
Emotional Aspect	*Hot*	*Dry*
Irascible	1. Hopefulness 2. Courage; temerity[2] 3. Easily provoked to anger	Brooding Anger lasts some time
Duration	Short	Long[1]
Mental Capacity		
Intellectual power	Good	Imaginative
Power of observation	Good	
Capability, talent	Good, conspicuous	Memory good
Moral Aspects	Stern Virility of morals and manners Diligence Much flexibility of opinion[2]	Gentle
Ego Instinctive Drive	Love of good opinion Not easily perturbed or downcast	Takes things to heart
Movements and Gestures Dreams	Of warming oneself at a fire; sitting in the hot sun[3]	

1 In the case of the moist temperament, the duration of emotional disturbance is short.

2 These represent negative or weak aspects.

3 In the case of a cold temperament, the dreams are of being in the cold, out in the snow or of being immersed in cold water. In short, the character of the visual images in the dream is related to the character of the dominant humour, partly because the dream varies with the state of the "breath" at the time.

11 Evidence of the Four Primary Intemperaments

Evidence	Hot	Cold	Moist	Dry
Morbid states to which there is a tendency.	Inflammatory conditions becoming febrile	Fevers related to the serous humour Rheumatism	Same as Cold	Evidence
	Loss of vigor			
Functional power	Deficient energy	Deficient digestive power	Difficult digestion	Evidence
Subjective sensations	Bitter taste in the mouth		Mucoid salivation	Evidence
	Excessive thirst	Lack of desire for fluids		
	Sense of burning at cardiac orifice		Sleepiness	Insomnia, wakefulness
Physical signs	Pulse extremely quick and frequent; approaching the weak type with in lassitude	Flaccid joints	Diarrhea Swollen eyelids	Rough skin Spare habit (acquired, not inborn)
Foods and medicines	Calefacients are all harmful,	Infrigidants are all harmful	Moist articles of diet harmful	Dry regimen harmful
	Infrigidants benefit	Calefacients benefit		Humectants beneficial[1]
Relation to weather	Worse in Summer	Worse in Winter		Bad in Autumn

1 Hot water, rarefied oils are beneficial to the dry temperament and are avidly taken up.

12 Sleep quiet, uninterrupted, and followed, on waking, by cheerfulness, and a contented mind.

13 Therefore no conscious feeling of digestion or discomfort of any kind. Micturition painless, the urine not feeling hot, having an odor neither sweet nor sour, amber-colored and forming no deposit. Defecation without soiling the skin, the feces firm, but not hard. The appetite according to genuine hunger and for natural foods, thirst only for water. Mouth closed when breathing. Adaptability to climate and season (*Chahar maqala*).

14 The modern term "hypertension" is covered by the old term of plethora or repletion. The correspondence is verified by some of its symptoms. Thus hemorrhagic phenomena occur—in the nose, retina, cerebrum, meninges, labyrinth, the skin and as hematuria and hemetemesis simulating organic disease. Hypertension causes fatigue of the heart shown by: dyspnea, palpitation, quick pulse, anginal attacks, nocturnal pseudo-asthma, *brut de galop*.

15 One or two of the data given (under general physique: on the hair; the surface veins) are from Rhazes. Note the patient at rest (in repose) and in activity (gestures, attitude). Note that the signs of his temperament are accentuated when he is ill. The type of reaction to infection is determined by his temperament.

16 Evidence which show Which of the Humours is Dominant

Evidence	*Sanguineous*	*Serous*	*Choleric*	*Atrabilious*
Aspect: General Physique	Good	Effeminate; bones slender; joints well-covered	Lean; joints large	Emaciated
Color	Ruddy	Unduly pale	Yellow tinge in and conjunctiva	Dusky; whole body seems dark, hairy
Feel of body	Flesh firm	Soft and cool		Flesh hard
State of skin	Reddens on rubbing; furuncles			Skin rough; liable to dark eruptions; intractable ulcers.
Hair			Hairy	
Surface veins	Full	Absent on truck. Constricted	Thick and hard	Hairy

Vegetative Drives

Mouth	Liability to pustules	Abundant sticky saliva	Bitter taste	Sense of burning at mouth of stomach
Tongue	Red		Rough, dry	
Nostrils			Rough, dry	
Pulse			Soft, tends to be slow, infrequent	
Urine			White	Dark colored or black; dense
Feces				

Sensitive Drives

Evidence	*Sanguineous*	*Serous*	*Choleric*	*Atrabilious*
Special Senses: taste	Unusual sweetness in mouth, senses dull		Bitter taste	Sense of burning at mouth of stomach
Appetite for food			Poor	Depraved
Appetite for fluid		Absent unless salt is taken esp. for elderly	Thirsty	
Muscular tone	Weariness not accounted for by exertion	Flaccidity of limbs		
Dreams				
Movements (gestures)	Yawning, stretching, slow reaction time, continual drowsiness	Somnolence, laziness, tiredness	Hebetude.	Sense of anxiety; wakefulness.

Abnormal Drives

Nausea	Present		Present	
Vomiting			Yellow-green bile, acrid flux	
Goose flesh			Needle-pricks	
Headache	Sense of weight in back of eyes and temple			
Others	Blood flows out readily from nose, anus, gums	Weak digestion and acid eructations	Severe diarrhea	Splenic disorders often occur, also morphoea; evil ulcers

Preceding Factors

Diet, occupations, locality living in, habits, season of year, date of last venesection, previous temperament

17 The subject of obstructions is capable of great expansion. The symptoms differ: (1) With each of the humours: (i) Thus serous humour obstructions are manifested as oedema of the glottis, odema of the lung, nasopharyngeal hypersecretion, odema of the kidney tissue, of the blood itself, vomiting, diarrhea, headache (too much cerebro-spinal fluid), convulsions, delirium, coma, Cheyne-Stokes respiration, amaurosis. (ii) With the different substances, thus in nephritis, obstruction of the channels in the skin prevents the wastes leaving the body by that route with consequent manifestation as arthritis, anginas, otitis, etc.

(iii) With the atom groups, thus obstruction to the outlet of nitrogen (azotemia) manifests as hypertension, vomiting, diarrhea, sialorrhea, stomatitis, parotitis, retinitis, anemia of plasmatic type, arthralgia, fibrillar tremors, coma, loss of appetite for meats. Viewing diseases in this way, the important thing is to find both site of obstruction and substance or atom-groups concerned. (2) The symptoms may be monosyndromic or polysyndromic. (3) There may be obstruction to the flow of "breath." (4) The pores which may become obstructed vary in size from that of the orifices of the body down to the smallest channels, whether visible to the naked eye or only with the microscope or whether sub-microscopic or ultra-microscopic. The pores vary in shape and consistence, resilience, elasticity, distensibility. Fluids may traverse them in both directions, but when there is obstruction, they may be able to pass only in one direction or not at all.

NOTES

Notes

Printed in the USA
CPSIA information can be obtained
at www.ICGtesting.com
JSHW022100030823
45883JS00002B/110

9 781567 447897